Macaroni

TAKE CHARG
THE MOST AU
CALORIE C

THE
CORINNE T. NETZER
1999
CALORIE COUNTER

If you're keeping track of calories, there's no better, more accurate portable guide than the book that has helped millions of calorie-conscious consumers make informed choices about the foods they eat.

Whether you're cruising the supermarket aisles, bringing home takeout for an easy meal, or feeling like a treat, here's the slim, handy reference that takes the guesswork out of calorie counting. Discover up-to-date calorie counts for the newest brand names as well as old favorites in this latest edition of America's #1 calorie counter. Pocket-size for easy portability, updated annually for true accuracy, *The Corinne T. Netzer 1999 Calorie Counter* gives you the information you need—at home, at work, wherever you go—to eat wisely and well.

THE
CORINNE T. NETZER
1999
CALORIE COUNTER

Corinne T. Netzer

A Dell Book

Published by
Dell Publishing
a division of
Bantam Doubleday Dell Publishing Group, Inc.
1540 Broadway
New York, New York 10036

The trademark Dell® is registered in the U.S. Patent and Trademark
Office.

ISBN: 0-440-22584-1

Printed in the United States of America

Published simultaneously in Canada

November 1998

10 9 8 7 6 5 4 3 2 1

OPM

Introduction

The Corinne T. Netzer Calorie Counter has been compiled with a twofold purpose: as an annual to keep you up-to-date with many of the changes made by the food industry, and to provide a handy, put-in-purse-or-pocket volume.

My books *The Complete Book of Food Counts, The Corinne T. Netzer Dieter's Diary,* and *The Brand-Name Calorie Counter* are much larger in size and scope, and are therefore much less portable. However, *this book contains more products than any other book of its size!*

To keep this book concise yet comprehensive, I have grouped together listings of the same manufacturer whenever possible. Many brand-name yogurts, for example, are listed as "all fruit flavors." Therefore, instead of filling three pages with individual flavors of yogurt, all with identical calorie counts, I have been able to use the extra space for many other products. And for many basic foods and beverages (such as oil, milk, and alcoholic beverages), I have used generic listings, rather than include the numerous brands with the same or similar caloric values.

Finally, in the process of updating this edition, it was necessary to eliminate many previous listings and brands to accommodate new products and different brands. If you do not find a specific brand-name food that was listed in a previous edition of this book, *this does not necessarily mean that the food product is no longer available.* Also, since food producers are constantly revising and improving products, the caloric count of your favorite food may have changed even if the description of the product hasn't. Be sure to check for updated entries.

This book contains data from individual producers and

manufacturers and from the United States government. It contains the most current information available as we go to press.

Good luck—and good eating.

C.T.N.

Abbreviations

approx. . . . . approximately
cont. . . . . container
diam. . . . . diameter
fl. . . . . fluid
lb. . . . . pound(s)
oz. . . . . ounce(s)
pkg. . . . . package
pkt. . . . . packet
tbsp. . . . . tablespoon(s)
tsp. . . . . teaspoon(s)
w/ . . . . with

Symbols

   . . . . inch
< . . . . less than
* . . . . prepared according to
basic package directions

Note: Brand-name foods and restaurants listed in italics denote registered trademarks.

THE
CORINNE T. NETZER
1999
CALORIE COUNTER

A

Acerola juice, fresh, 6 fl. oz. 36
Acorn squash:
(Frieda's), ¾ cup, 3 oz. 35
baked, cubed, ½ cup 57
Adobo *(Durkee),* ¼ tsp. 0
Adzuki beans, dry *(Arrowhead Mills),* ¼ cup 160
Alfalfa sprouts:
(Arrowhead Mills), 1 cup 30
(Jonathan's), 1 cup 25
Alfredo sauce:
canned *(Progresso* Authentic), ½ cup 300
canned, three cheese *(Lawry's),* 3 tbsp. 70
refrigerated *(Contadina),* ¼ cup 180
refrigerated *(Contadina* Light), ¼ cup 80
Alfredo sauce mix:
(Knorr), ⅓ pkg. 60
(Spice Islands), ½ pkg. 45
seasoning *(Lawry's),* 1½ tbsp. 35
Allspice, 1 tsp. 5
Almond, shelled:
(Dole), 1 oz. 170
dried, slivered, 1 cup 795
honey-roasted *(Planters),* 1 oz. 160
slivered *(Planters Gold Measure),* 2-oz. pkg. 340
tamari-roasted *(Eden),* 1 oz. 170
Almond butter *(Roaster Fresh),* 1 oz. 184
Almond paste *(Solo),* 2 tbsp. 180
Amaranth entree, canned *(Health Valley* Fast Menu),
   1 cup 160
Anasazi beans *(Arrowhead Mills),* ¼ cup 150
Anchovy, canned, in olive oil *(King Oscar),* 6 fillets,
   .5 oz. 25

Anchovy paste *(Reese),* 1 tbsp. 30
Angel-hair pasta entree, frozen *(Smart Ones),* 9 oz. . . . 170
Anise seed, 1 tsp. 7
Appaloosa beans, dry *(Frieda's),* ½cup 120
Apple:
fresh *(Frieda's* Lady Apple), 5 oz. 80
fresh, peeled, sliced, ½ cup 31
canned, ½ cup, except as noted:
    baked, Dutch *(Lucky Leaf/Musselman's)* 170
    fried *(Apple Time/Lucky Leaf)* 170
    sliced *(Lucky Leaf/Musselman's)* 50
    sliced *(White House)* 100
    spiced, whole *(Comstock/Wilderness),* 1 piece 35
    spiced rings *(Comstock/Wilderness),* 2 rings 25
    spiced rings *(S&W),* 2 rings 25
dried *(Sonoma),* 1.4 oz. 110
dried, chips *(Smart Snackers),* .75 oz. 70
dried, sliced *(Del Monte),* ⅓ cup, 1.4 oz. 80
Apple, escalloped:
canned *(White House),* ½ cup 160
frozen *(Stouffer's),* 6 oz. 180
Apple butter, 1 tbsp.:
(Apple Time/Lucky Leaf/Musselman's) 30
(Dutch Girl/Mary Ellen) 35
(Smucker's Simply Fruit) 40
all flavors *(Smucker's)* 45
spread *(Apple Time)* 25
Apple chips, all varieties *(Seneca),* 1 oz. 140
Apple drink blends, 8 fl. oz., except as noted:
all flavors, except peach-kiwi/plum *(Veryfine*
    Quenchers) 120
berry burst *(Dole)* 120
berry pear *(Tropicana Twister)* 140
cherry squeeze *(Snapple)* 120
cranberry *(Dole),* 10 fl. oz. 160
peach-kiwi or peach-plum *(Veryfine Quenchers)* 130
punch *(Minute Maid)* 120
raspberry-blackberry *(Tropicana Twister)* 130
Apple fritters, frozen *(Mrs. Paul's),* 2 pieces 260

Apple juice, 8 fl. oz., except as noted:

(Apple & Eve) 110
(Apple Time/Lincoln/Lucky Leaf Regular/Cider) 120
(Apple Time/Lucky Leaf/Musselman's), 5.5 fl. oz. 80
(Mott's Natural) 120
(Musselman's Regular/Natural/Cider) 120
(Musselman's Premium Natural) 130
(R.W. Knudsen Clear/Aseptic) 110
(R.W. Knudsen Natural/Organic/Gravenstein) 120
(Red Cheek) 120
(S&W) 120
(Snapple), 12 fl. oz. 180
(Snapple Crisp), 10 fl. oz. 140
(Veryfine) 120
cider, sparkling *(Apple Time/Lucky Leaf/Musselman's)* . 150
frozen* *(Minute Maid)* 110
spiced *(Apple & Eve* Cider & Spice) 110
Apple juice blends, 8 fl. oz.:
all blends, except cherry cider *(R.W. Knudsen)* 120
apricot *(Tree Top* Fiber Rich) 160
cherry cider, bottled or frozen* *(R.W. Knudsen)* 130
cranberry *(Apple & Eve)* 120
cranberry, frozen* *(Tree Top)* 130
grape *(Juicy Juice)* 130
grape, bottled or frozen* *(Tree Top)* 130
raspberry *(Tree Top* Box) 120
raspberry, frozen* *(Tree Top)* 110
Apple pastry (see also specific listings):
dumpling, frozen *(Pepperidge Farm),* 1 piece 290
pocket *(Tastykake),* 1 piece 380
Applesauce, ½ cup:
(Lincoln) 90
(Mott's/Mott's Chunky) 110
(Mott's Cinnamon) 120
(S&W Gravenstein) 90
(Seneca Regular/Cinnamon/McIntosh) 100
unsweetened *(Lucky Leaf* Regular/Cinnamon) 50
unsweetened *(S&W* Gravenstein) 50
unsweetened *(Santa Cruz* Regular/Gravenstein) 45

Apricot:
fresh, whole, 3 medium, 12 per lb. 51
canned *(Del Monte Lite)*, ½ cup 60
canned, in juice *(Libby's Lite)*, ½ cup 60
canned, in heavy syrup *(S&W)*, ½ cup 110
dried *(Dole Sun Giant)*, 6 pieces, 1.4 oz. 90
dried *(Sonoma)*, 1.4 oz. 120
sun-dried *(Del Monte)*, ⅓ cup, 1.4 oz. 80
Apricot juice *(Ceres)*, 8 fl. oz. 120
Apricot nectar, 8 fl. oz.:
(Libby's/Kern's) 150
(R.W. Knudsen) 120
Artichoke, globe:
fresh, boiled, 10.6-oz. choke 60
canned, bottoms *(S&W)*, 3 pieces 25
canned, hearts, in brine *(Progresso)*, 2 pieces 30
frozen, hearts, 9-oz. pkg. 96
Artichoke, Jerusalem, see "Jerusalem artichoke"
Artichoke appetizer, marinated:
(Contorno Caponata di Carciofi), ⅓ cup 130
marinated *(Progresso)*, 2 oz. 60
in olive oil *(Goya)*, 3 oz. 210
Artichoke paste *(Cucina Aromatica)*, 1 oz. 125
Arugula, trimmed *(Frieda's)*, 3.5 oz. 23
Asparagus:
fresh, raw *(Dole)*, 5 spears 25
fresh, boiled, 4 spears, ½ -diam. base 14
canned *(S&W* Blended), 6 pieces 15
canned *(S&W* Colossal), 3 pieces 10
canned, all varieties *(Del Monte)*, ½ cup 20
canned, spears *(Green Giant/LeSueur)*, 4.5 oz. 20
frozen, cuts *(Birds Eye)*, ½ cup 25
frozen, spears *(Birds Eye)*, 3 oz. 20
Asparagus, pickled, in jars *(Hogue Farms)*, 3 spears,
   1.1 oz. 10
Au jus gravy, ¼ cup:
(Franco-American) 10
mix* *(Durkee/French's)* 5
mix* *(Knorr)* 15

Au jus seasoning mix *(Durkee/French's* Roasting Bag),
   1/8 pkg. 10
Avocado, California:
(Dole), 1/5 medium, 1.1 oz. 20
pureed, 1/2 cup 204
Avocado dip *(Nalley/Nalley* Guacamole), 2 tbsp. 120

B

Bacon, cooked, 2 slices, except as noted:
(Boar's Head) 60
(Hormel Layout Pack/Hormel Layout Pack Low Salt) 80
(John Morrell Hardwood Smoked) 100
(Oscar Mayer/Oscar Mayer Center Cut/Lower Sodium) . . 60
(Oscar Mayer Thick), 1 slice 60
(Wilson Hickory Smoked) 80
turkey, see "Turkey bacon"
Bacon, Canadian *(Boar's Head),* 2 oz. 70
"Bacon," vegetarian, frozen:
(Morningstar Farms Breakfast Strips), 2 strips 60
(Worthington Stripples), 2 strips 60
Bacon bits:
(Oscar Mayer/Oscar Mayer Pieces), 1 tbsp. 25
imitation *(Bac'n Pieces),* 1½ tbsp. 30
imitation *(Bac*Os),* 1½ tbsp. 30
Bacon dip, 2 tbsp.:
horseradish *(Heluva* Good) 60
horseradish *(Heluva* Good Free) 25
onion *(Breakstone's)* 60
onion *(Nalley)* 110
Bagel, 1 piece:
plain *(Thomas')* 150
plain or blueberry *(Awrey's),* 4-oz. piece 280
plain or cinnamon raisin *(Awrey's),* 2.6-oz. piece 200
cinnamon raisin *(Awrey's),* 4-oz. piece 270
cinnamon raisin or egg *(Thomas')* 160
mini *(Awrey's)* 100
multigrain or onion *(Thomas')* 150
Bagel, frozen, plain *(Sara Lee),* 1 piece 220
Baked beans, canned, ½ cup:
(Allens) 150
(Campbell's New England Style) 180

Baked beans *(cont.)*

(Hunt's Country Kettle) 150
(Hunt's Mix and Serve) 125
(Hunt's Special Recipe) 185
(S&W Brick Oven) 160
(Van Camp Fat Free) 130
(Van Camp Original/Premium) 140
bacon and brown sugar:
    (Bush's Best Original/Homestyle) 150
    (Campbell's) 170
    (S&W) 140
    spiced *(Bush's* Best Bold & Spicy) 120
barbecue *(Campbell's/Campbell's* Old Fashioned) 170
barbecue, Texas style *(S&W)* 140
brown sugar *(Van Camp)* 170
chili, see "Chili beans" and "Mexican beans"
hickory, sweet and bacon *(Van Camp)* 140
honey *(Health Valley/Health Valley* No Salt) 110
honey mustard *(S&W)* 130
maple sugar *(S&W)* 150
w/pork:
    (Campbell's) 130
    (Crest Top) 130
    (Green Giant/Joan of Arc) 120
    (Hunt's) 130
    (Hunt's Homestyle) 155
    (Stokely Sugar) 150
    (Stokely Tomato) 140
    (Van Camp) 110
    (Wagon Master/Trappey's) 110
    w/jalapeño *(Trappey's)* 130
ranch *(Open Range)* 125
Southern style, w/sautéed onion *(Van Camp)* 145
vegetarian *(Eden* Organic) 150
vegetarian *(Stokely)* 140
vegetarian *(Van Camp)* 110
vegetarian, brown sugar sauce *(Stokely)* 150
Baking mix (see also "Biscuit mix"):
(Bisquick), ⅓ cup 170
(Bisquick Reduced Fat), ⅓ cup 150

all-purpose *(Arrowhead Mills)*, ¼ cup 140
Balsam pear *(Frieda's* Bittermelon), 1 cup, 3 oz. 15
Bamboo shoots:
fresh, boiled, drained, ½ slices, ½ cup 8
canned, drained *(La Choy/Chun King),* 2 tbsp. 3
Banana, fresh:
(Dole), 1 medium 120
1 medium, 8¾ long 105
burro, manzano, nino, or red *(Frieda's),* 5 oz. 130
Banana, baking, see "Plantain"
Banana, dried:
(Frieda's), 1 piece 130
(Sonoma), 2 pieces 140
Banana squash *(Frieda's),* ¾ cup, 3 oz. 30
Barbecue dip *(Heluva* Good), 2 tbsp. 60
Barbecue sauce, 2 tbsp., except as noted:
(Heinz Thick & Rich Old Fashioned) 40
(Hunt's Original) 40
(Hunt's Original Bold) 45
(Hunt's Original Light) 25
(KC Masterpiece Original) 60
(Lea & Perrins Original/Bold & Spicy) 50
all varieties *(Healthy Choice)* 25
all varieties, except honey and spice *(Open Pit* Thick
    and Tangy) 50
all varieties, except sweet and sour *(Open Pit).* 50
Dijon, mild *(Hunt's)* 40
garlic and herb *(Lea & Perrins)* 40
hickory *(Hunt's)* 40
hickory *(Hunt's* Bold) 45
hickory and brown sugar *(Hunt's)* 75
hickory smoke *(Kraft/Kraft* Hot) 40
hickory smoke, w/onion bits *(Kraft)* 50
honey *(Heinz* Thick & Rich) 45
honey *(Kraft)* 50
honey *(Kraft Thick'N Spicy)* 60
honey Dijon *(KC Masterpiece)* 50
honey hickory *(Hunt's)* 55
honey mustard *(Hunt's)* 45
honey and spice *(Open Pit* Thick and Tangy) 45

Barbecue sauce *(cont.)*

hot *(Kraft)* 40
hot and spicy *(Hunt's)* 45
Italian *(Porino's)* 40
jalapeño or Kansas City style *(Maull's)* 60
mesquite *(Hunt's)* 40
mild *(Hunt's)* 40
Oriental *(House of Tsang* Hong Kong), 1 tsp. 10
Oriental, pork *(House of Tsang)* 90
sweet and sour *(Open Pit)* 45
teriyaki *(Hunt's)* 45

Barley:

dry, pearled *(Arrowhead Mills)*, ¼ cup 170
cooked, pearled, 1 cup 193

Basil:

fresh, 5 medium leaves or 2 tbsp. chopped 1
dried, ground, 1 tsp. 4

Baskin-Robbins:

ice cream, deluxe, ½ cup:

banana strawberry 130
Baseball Nut or black walnut 160
butter pecan, old fashion 160
Butterfinger 160
cherries jubilee 140
chocolate 150
chocolate, world class 160
chocolate almond 180
chocolate chip or chocolate chip mint 150
chocolate chip cookie dough 170
chocolate fudge 160
chocolate mousse royale 170
chocolate raspberry truffle 180
cookies 'n cream 170
egg nog 150
Everyone's Favorite Candy Bar 170
French vanilla 160
fudge brownie 170
German chocolate cake 180
gold medal ribbon 150
Heath bar, chunky 170

jamoca 140
jamoca, almond fudge 160
lemon custard 150
Oregon blackberry 140
peach, pumpkin pie, or very berry strawberry 130
peanut butter 'n chocolate 180
pistachio-almond 170
pralines 'n cream 160
Quarterback Crunch 160
Reese's peanut butter 180
rocky road 170
rum raisin 140
strawberry cheesecake 150
Triple Chocolate Passion 180
vanilla 140
white chocolate, winter 150
ice cream, light, ½ cup:
  caramel apple à la mode or espresso 'n cream 100
  Maui Brownie Madness or *Perils of Praline* 140
ice cream, fat free, ½ cup:
  berry cheesecake or jamoca swirl 110
  Check-It-Out-Cherry 100
ice cream, no sugar added, ½ cup:
  Call Me Nuts 110
  cherry cordial or Thin Mint 100
  Mad About Chocolate 100
  pineapple coconut 90
ices, sherbets, and sorbets, ½ cup:
  daiquiri or watermelon ice 110
  The Mask ice 120
  orange, rainbow, or blue raspberry sherbet 120
  raspberry lemon sorbet, pink 120
Bass (see also "Sea bass"), meat only, 4 oz.:
freshwater, baked or broiled 166
striped, baked or broiled 141
Bay leaf, dried, crumbled, 1 tsp. 5
Bean dip, 2 tbsp.:
(Chi-Chi's Fiesta) 35
(Fritos) 40
(Old Dutch) 30

Bean dip *(cont.)*
(Old El Paso) 20
jalapeño *(Fritos)* 35
Bean dip mix, black or Mexican *(Knorr),* 1 tsp. 10
Bean loaf, frozen *(Natural Touch),* 1 slice 160
Bean salad, in jars:
deli style *(S&W),* ½ cup 80
marinated *(S&W),* ½ cup 70
three bean *(Green Giant),* ½ cup 90
Bean sauce, brown, spicy *(House of Tsang),* 1 tsp. 15
Bean sprouts, see "Sprouts" and specific listings
Beans, see specific bean listings
Beef, choice, meat only, trimmed to ¼ fat, except as
  noted, 4 oz.:
brisket, whole, braised, lean w/fat 437
brisket, whole, braised, lean only 274
chuck, arm pot roast, braised, lean w/fat 395
chuck, arm pot roast, braised, lean only 255
chuck, blade roast, braised, lean w/fat 412
chuck, blade roast, braised, lean only 298
flank steak, trimmed to 0 fat, broiled, lean only 256
ground, broiled, medium, extra lean 290
ground, broiled, medium, lean 308
ground, broiled, medium, regular 328
porterhouse steak, broiled, lean w/fat 346
porterhouse steak, broiled, lean only 247
rib, whole, roasted, lean w/fat 426
rib, whole, roasted, lean only 276
round, bottom, braised, lean w/fat 322
round, bottom, braised, lean only 249
round, eye of, roasted, lean w/fat 273
round, eye of, roasted, lean only 198
round, tip, roasted, lean w/fat 280
round, tip, roasted, lean only 213
round, top, broiled, lean w/fat 254
round, top, broiled, lean only 214
sirloin, top, broiled, lean w/fat 305
sirloin, top, broiled, lean only 229
sirloin, top, fried, lean w/fat 370
sirloin, top, fried, lean only 270

T-bone steak, broiled, lean w/fat 338
T-bone steak, broiled, lean only 243
tenderloin, broiled, lean w/fat 345
tenderloin, broiled, lean only 252
top loin, broiled, lean w/fat 338
top loin, broiled, lean only 243
Beef, corned (see also "Beef lunch meat"):
brisket, cooked, 4 oz. 285
canned *(Goya)*, 2 oz. 120
Beef, dried, sliced *(Hormel)*, 1 oz. 50
"Beef," vegetarian (see also " 'Hamburger,'
   vegetarian"):
canned:
   (Worthington Savory Slices), 3 slices 150
   (Worthington Prime Stakes), 1 piece 140
   (Worthington Vegetable Steaks), 2 slices 80
   stew *(Worthington* Country), 1 cup 210
frozen:
   (Worthington Meatless), ⅜ slice 110
   corned *(Worthington* Slices), 4 slices 140
   smoked *(Worthington* Sliced), 6 slices 120
Beef dinner, frozen:
broccoli Beijing *(Healthy Choice)*, 11 oz. 300
and broccoli *(Swanson)*, 1 pkg. 350
and broccoli *(Swanson Hungry-Man)*, 1 pkg. 490
chicken-fried steak *(Banquet* Extra Helping), 16 oz. 820
chicken-fried steak, w/gravy *(Swanson)*, 1 pkg. 460
country fried steak *(Swanson Hungry-Man)*, 1 pkg. 660
enchilada, see "Enchilada dinner"
and gravy *(Swanson)*, 1 pkg. 370
mesquite w/barbeque sauce *(Healthy Choice)*, 11 oz. . . . 320
patty, charbroiled, gravy and *(Morton)*, 9 oz. 310
w/peppers, Cantonese *(Healthy Choice)*, 11.5 oz. 270
pot roast, Yankee *(Banquet* Extra Helping), 14.5 oz. 410
pot roast, Yankee *(Healthy Choice)*, 11 oz. 290
pot roast, Yankee *(Swanson)*, 1 pkg. 250
pot roast, Yankee *(Swanson Hungry-Man)*, 1 pkg. 360
roast, sandwich, smothered *(Swanson)*, 1 pkg. 350
Salisbury steak:
   (Banquet Extra Helping), 16.5 oz. 780

Beef dinner, Salisbury steak *(cont.)*

(Healthy Choice), 11 oz.	310
(Healthy Choice Traditional), 11.5 oz.	330
(Swanson), 1 pkg.	340
(Swanson Hungry-Man), 1 pkg.	610
con queso *(Patio)*, 11 oz.	390
gravy and *(Morton)*, 9 oz.	310
sirloin, chopped, w/gravy *(Swanson)*, 1 pkg.	380
sirloin tips *(Swanson Hungry-Man)*, 1 pkg.	440
sirloin tips, w/noodles *(Swanson)*, 1 pkg.	290
Stroganoff *(Healthy Choice)*, 11 oz.	310
tips, traditional *(Healthy Choice)*, 11.25 oz.	280

Beef entree, canned (see also "Beef hash"):

chow mein *(La Choy/Chun King* Bi-Pack), 1 cup	80
pepper, Oriental *(La Choy/Chun King* Bi-Pack), 1 cup	100
pepper, Oriental, w/noodles *(La Choy* Bi-Pack), 1 cup	160
pot roast *(Dinty Moore American Classics)*, 10 oz.	210
Salisbury steak *(Dinty Moore American Classics)*, 10 oz.	310
stew *(Dinty Moore* Can/Cup), 7½ oz.	190
stew *(Dinty Moore American Classics)*, 10 oz.	260
stew *(Hormel* Micro Cup), 7½ oz.	180
stew *(Hunt's* Homestyle), 1 cup	155
stew, burger *(Dinty Moore* Hearty Cup), 7½ oz.	240

Beef entree, frozen:

chicken-fried *(Banquet)*, 10 oz.	420
chipped, creamed *(Banquet* Topper), 4-oz. bag	120
chipped, creamed *(Stouffer's)*, 4.4 oz.	160
enchilada, see "Enchilada entree"	
ground, w/rice *(Goya)*, 1 pkg.	860
macaroni *(Healthy Choice)*, 8.5 oz.	210
mesquite, w/rice *(Lean Cuisine* Cafe Classics), 9 oz.	280
noodles w/ *(Freezer Queen* Family), 1 cup, 8.5 oz.	200
Oriental *(The Budget Gourmet* Light), 9 oz.	250
Oriental *(Lean Cuisine)*, 9¼ oz.	240
patty:	
charbroiled, mushroom gravy and *(Banquet* Family), 1 patty w/gravy	230
w/country-style vegetables *(Banquet)*, 9.5 oz.	310
grilled peppercorn *(Healthy Choice)*, 9 oz.	220

onion gravy and *(Banquet* Family), 1 patty w/gravy . 180
western style *(Banquet)*, 9.5 oz. 380
pepper, Oriental *(La Choy)*, 1 cup 150
pepper steak *(Stouffer's)*, 10½ oz. 330
pepper steak *(Weight Watchers)*, 10 oz. 240
pepper steak Oriental *(Healthy Choice)*, 9.5 oz. 250
pie *(Banquet)*, 7-oz. pie 400
pie *(Swanson)*, 1 pkg. 415
pie *(Swanson Hungry-Man)*, 1 pkg. 660
pot roast, and gravy *(Marie Callender)*, 1 cup 260
pot roast, w/potato *(Stouffer's* Homestyle), 8⅞ oz. . . . 250
pot roast, Yankee *(Banquet)*, 9.4 oz. 230
roast *(Healthy Choice* Hearty Handfuls), 6.1 oz. 310
Salisbury steak:
    (Banquet), 9.5 oz. 380
    w/gravy, mashed potato *(Swanson* Lunch and
      More), 1 pkg. 330
    gravy and *(Banquet* Toppers), 5-oz. bag 210
    gravy, brown, and *(Banquet* Family), 1 patty w/gravy . 230
    grilled *(Weight Watchers)*, 8.5 oz. 260
    w/macaroni and cheese *(Lean Cuisine)*, 9.5 oz. 290
    w/macaroni and cheese *(Stouffer's* Homestyle),
      9⅝ oz. 350
    sirloin *(The Budget Gourmet* Light), 9 oz. 240
    sirloin *(Marie Callender)*, 14 oz. 550
sandwich, see "Beef sandwich"
sliced *(Banquet)*, 9 oz. 270
sliced, brown gravy and *(Banquet* Family), 2 slices
    w/gravy 100
sliced, gravy and *(Banquet* Topper), 4-oz. bag 70
sliced, gravy and *(Freezer Queen* Family), ⅔ cup,
    4.9 oz. 80
steak patty, grilled peppercorn *(Healthy Choice)*, 9 oz. . . 220
stew, hearty *(Banquet* Family), 1 cup, 8.7 oz. 160
Stroganoff *(The Budget Gourmet* Light), 8.75 oz. 290
Stroganoff *(Stouffer's)*, 9¾ oz. 390
tips, Français *(Healthy Choice)*, 9.5 oz. 280
tips, in mushroom sauce *(Marie Callender)*, 13.6 oz. . . . 430
Beef gravy, canned, ¼ cup:
(Franco-American) 30

Beef gravy *(cont.)*
(Franco-American Fat Free) 20
hearty *(Pepperidge Farm)* 25
slow-roasted *(Franco-American)* 25
Beef hash, canned, 1 cup, except as noted:
(Broadcast Morning Classics Original) 240
corned beef:
   (Dinty Moore Cup), 7½ oz. 200
   (Goya) 410
   (Libby's) 490
   (Mary Kitchen) 390
roast beef *(Libby's)* 460
roast beef *(Mary Kitchen)* 390
Beef lunch meat (see also "Bologna," etc.), 2 oz.:
corned *(Black Bear)* 60
corned *(Healthy Choice)* 60
corned, brisket *(Boar's Head)* 80
corned, round *(Healthy Deli)* 80
roast *(Hormel)* 60
roast *(Hormel* Top Round) 50
roast *(Hormel Light & Lean 97)* 60
roast, Italian or seasoned *(Healthy Deli)* 70
roast, plain, Cajun or Italian style *(Healthy Choice)* 60
roast, round, all varieties *(Boar's Head)* 90
Beef pie, see "Beef entree, frozen"
Beef sandwich, frozen, 1 piece:
barbecue *(Hormel Quick Meal)* 360
barbecue *(Hot Pockets)* 340
cheddar *(Hot Pockets)* 360
cheeseburger *(Hormel Quick Meal)* 400
cheeseburger, bacon *(Hormel Quick Meal)* 440
cheeseburger, chili *(Hormel Quick Meal)* 450
fajita *(Hot Pockets)* 360
hamburger *(Hormel Quick Meal)* 350
roast beef *(Healthy Choice Hearty Handfuls)* 310
steak, cheese *(Deli Stuffs)* 370
steak, Philly *(Healthy Choice Hearty Handfuls)* 290
steak, Philly, and cheese *(Croissant Pockets)* 370
Beef spread, roast *(Underwood)*, ¼ cup 140

Beer:

regular, 12 fl. oz. 146
light, 12 fl. oz. 100
Beet, ½ cup, except as noted:
fresh, boiled, 2 medium, 2 diam., 3.5 oz. 44
canned, all varieties, in water *(Seneca)* 40
canned, all varieties, except Harvard *(Green Giant)* 35
canned, whole, baby *(LeSueur)* 35
canned, whole or sliced *(Del Monte)* 35
canned, whole, sliced, or julienne *(S&W)* 30
canned, Harvard *(Green Giant)*, ⅓ cup 60
canned, Harvard *(Greenwood)* 100
canned, pickled *(S&W)*, 1 oz. 15
canned, pickled, all varieties *(Greenwood)*, 1.1 oz. 25
canned, pickled, crinkle style *(Del Monte)* 80
Beet greens, boiled, drained, 1 pieces, ½ cup 20
Berry drink, 8 fl. oz.:
(After the Fall Oregon) 100
citrus *(Five Alive)* 110
nectar *(Santa Cruz)* 110
punch *(Minute Maid/Minute Maid* Box) 120
punch, red *(Tree Top* Juice Rivers Box) 130
Berry juice, 8 fl. oz.:
(Apple & Eve Nothin' But Juice) 120
(Juicy Juice) 130
(Veryfine Juice-Ups) 140
Biscuit:
(Awrey's Country), 1 piece 140
(Awrey's Round), 2 oz. 150
Biscuit, refrigerated, 1 piece, except as noted:
(Big Country Butter Tastin') 110
(Grands! Extra Rich) 220
(Grands! Butter Tastin') 200
(Grands! Butter Tastin' Reduced Fat) 190
all varieties *(Hungry Jack)* 100
butter, buttermilk, or country *(Pillsbury)*, 3 pieces 150
buttermilk *(1869 Brand)* 100
buttermilk *(Pillsbury* Tender Layer), 3 pieces 160
buttermilk, cinnamon raisin, extra fluffy, or Southern
　　style *(Grands!)* 200

Biscuit, refrigerated *(cont.)*
buttermilk or Southern style *(Big Country)* 110
flaky or homestyle *(Grands!)* 190
Biscuit, frozen, garlic-cheese *(Pepperidge Farm),*
 1 piece 170
Biscuit mix (see also "Baking mix"):
(Gold Medal Biscuit Mix), 2 biscuits* 180
buttermilk *(Martha White Bismix),* 1/2 cup* 160
Biscuit sandwich, breakfast, frozen, sausage, egg, and
 cheese *(Great Starts),* 1 pkg. 460
Black bean dishes, mix, 3/8 cup:
Jamaican, and brown rice *(Fantastic* One Pot Meals) . . . 140
zesty, and penne *(Fantastic* One Pot Meals) 150
Black bean sauce *(Ka•Me),* 1 tbsp. 10
Black beans (see also "Refried beans"):
dried *(Frieda's),* 1/3 cup, 3 oz. 120
dried, boiled, 1/2 cup 113
canned, 1/2 cup:
 (Green Giant/Joan of Arc) 100
 (Old El Paso) 130
 (Progresso) 110
 (Stokely) 110
 w/ginger and lemon *(Eden* Organic) 120
 regular or seasoned *(Allens/Trappey's)* 120
Blackberry:
fresh, trimmed, 1/2 cup 37
canned *(Allens),* 2/3 cup 60
canned, in syrup *(Comstock/Wilderness),* 1/2 cup 110
canned, in syrup *(Oregon),* 1/2 cup 120
frozen, unsweetened, 1/2 cup 49
Black-eyed peas (see also "Cowpeas"), canned,
 1/2 cup:
fresh shell *(Allens/East Texas Fair/Homefolks)* 120
fresh shell *(Goya* Cowpeas) 90
fresh shell *(Stokely)* 110
fresh shell, w/jalapeño *(Homefolks)* 120
dry *(Allens/East Texas Fair)* 110
dry *(Green Giant/Joan of Arc)* 90
dry, w/bacon *(Allens/Sunshine)* 105
dry, w/bacon *(Trappey's)* 120

dry, w/bacon and jalapeño *(Trappey's)* 110
Bloody Mary mixer *(V-8)*, 11.5 fl. oz. 70
Blue squash, Australian *(Frieda's)*, ¾ cup, 3 oz. 35
Blueberry:
fresh, ½ cup 41
canned, in syrup *(Oregon)*, ½ cup 110
canned, in heavy syrup *(Comstock/Wilderness)*, ½ cup . 110
canned, in heavy syrup *(S&W* Wild Maine), ⅓ cup . . 70
frozen, sweetened, ½ cup 94
dried *(Frieda's)*, ¼ cup, 1.4 oz. 140
Blueberry syrup *(R.W. Knudsen)*, ¼ cup 150
Bluefish, meat only, baked or broiled, 4 oz. 180
Bologna (see also "Turkey bologna"):
(Black Bear German Brand), 2 oz. 160
(Boar's Head), 2 oz. 150
(Boar's Head 28% Lower Sodium), 2 oz. 150
(Healthy Deli Regular/German 95% Fat Free), 2 oz. 70
(John Morrell), 2 oz. 180
(Oscar Mayer), 1-oz. slice 90
beef *(Boar's Head)*, 2 oz. 150
beef *(Oscar Mayer)*, 1-oz. slice 90
beef *(Oscar Mayer* Light), 1-oz. slice 60
garlic *(Boar's Head)*, 2 oz. 150
"Bologna," vegetarian *(Worthington* Bolono), 3 slices . . 80
Bouillabaisse seasoning mix *(Knorr* Recipe), 1 tbsp. . . 20
Bouillon, 1 tsp. or cube, except as noted:
beef or chicken *(Herb-Ox/Herb-Ox* Instant) 10
beef or chicken *(Knorr)* 20
fish *(Knorr)*, ½ cube 10
onion *(MBT* Instant), 1 pkt. 15
vegetable *(Herb-Ox)* 10
vegetable, vegetarian *(Knorr)*, ½ cube 15
Bourguignonne seasoning *(Knorr)*, 1 tbsp. 35
Bow-tie pasta dishes, mix, 1 cup*:
cheese, Italian *(Lipton* Pasta & Sauce) 290
chicken primavera *(Lipton* Pasta & Sauce) 300
Bow-tie pasta entree, frozen:
Alfredo or marinara *(Marie Callender)*, 13 oz. 430
and chicken *(Lean Cuisine* Cafe Classics), 9.5 oz. 270

Bow-tie pasta entree *(cont.)*
and creamy tomato sauce *(Lean Cuisine Lunch
Classics)*, 9.5 oz. 290
and meat sauce *(Marie Callender)*, 13 oz. 480
Boysenberry, ½ cup:
fresh, see "Blackberry"
canned, in syrup *(Comstock/Wilderness)* 120
canned, in syrup *(Oregon)* 120
Boysenberry cider *(Heinke's)*, 8 fl. oz. 120
Bratwurst *(Jones Dairy Farm* Dinner), 1 cooked link . . . 230
Braunschweiger:
(Oscar Mayer), 1-oz. slice 100
light *(Boar's Head)*, 2 oz. 120
sliced *(Jones Dairy Farm)*, 1.2-oz. slice 110
sliced *(Jones Dairy Farm)*, 2 slices, 1.6 oz. 150
spread *(Oscar Mayer)*, 2 oz. 190
smoked *(Black Bear* Liverwurst), 2 oz. 180
w/bacon or onion *(Jones Dairy Farm* Chub), 2 oz. 150
Brazil nut, shelled, 1 oz., 6 large or 8 medium kernels . 186
Bread, 1 slice, except as noted:
(Arnold/Arnold Bran'nola Country) 90
bran, honey *(Pepperidge Farm)* 90
bran, whole *(Brownberry)* 60
cinnamon *(Brownberry)* 80
date nut *(Thomas')*, 1 oz. 80
French *(Arnold Francisco)*, 1 oz. 70
French *(Pepperidge Farm)*, ⅑ loaf 130
Italian *(Arnold Francisco)*, 2 slices 110
Italian *(Wonder* 20 oz.) 80
Italian, brown and serve *(Pepperidge Farm)*, ⅑ loaf . . . 130
Italian, light *(Arnold/Brownberry Bakery)*, 2 slices 80
mixed grain/multigrain:
  (Healthy Choice) 60
  5, sprouted *(Shiloh Farms/Shiloh Farms* No Salt) 90
  7 *(Healthy Choice)* 80
  7 or 12 *(Roman Meal)* 70
  7, light *(Roman Meal)*, 2 slices 80
  7, white *(Arnold/Brownberry Bran'nola)* 90
  9 *(Pepperidge Farm)* 90
  12 *(Arnold Bran'nola)* 90

crunchy *(Pepperidge Farm)* 90
w/oat bran *(Roman Meal)* 70
whole *(Healthy Choice)* 80
whole *(Pepperidge Farm* 100%) 90
oat *(Brownberry Bran'nola)* 90
oat, crunchy, hearty *(Pepperidge Farm)* 100
oat bran, honey or honey nut *(Roman Meal)* 70
oatmeal *(Brownberry* Natural/Soft) 70
oatmeal *(Pepperidge Farm)* 80
oatmeal, light *(Pepperidge Farm)*, 3 slices 140
orange raisin *(Brownberry)* 70
pita or pocket:
　(Arnold), 2 oz. 140
　(Arnold), 3 oz. 210
　garlic *(Arnold)* 160
　onion *(Arnold)* 150
　wheat *(Arnold)*, 2 oz. 140
　wheat *(Arnold)*, 3 oz. 200
　white or wheat *(Arnold* 4), 1 oz. 70
potato *(Arnold* Country) 100
potato, hearty *(Pepperidge Farm* Russet) 90
pumpernickel *(Arnold/Arnold Levy's)* 80
pumpernickel, dark *(Pepperidge Farm)* 80
pumpernickel, rye *(Brownberry)* 70
pumpernickel or rye *(Pepperidge Farm* Party), 8 slices . 110
raisin *(Arnold Sunmaid)* 70
raisin cinnamon *(Arnold/Brownberry)* 70
rye *(Arnold* Deli/Dill) 80
rye *(Brownberry* Hearth) 90
rye, Dijon, thin *(Pepperidge Farm)*, 2 slices 100
rye, onion *(Arnold August Bros.)* 80
rye, seeded or unseeded *(Arnold August Bros.* 1 lb.) . . . 80
rye, seeded or unseeded *(Pepperidge Farm)* 80
rye, soft *(Arnold* Country) 70
rye, soft, seeded or unseeded *(Arnold Bakery)* 80
rye, thin *(Arnold Levy's Melba)*, 2 slices 90
sourdough *(Arnold Francisco)* 90
sourdough, brown and serve *(Arnold Francisco)*, 1 oz. . . 70
sourdough, light *(Arnold)*, 2 slices 80
sourdough, light *(Pepperidge Farm)*, 3 slices 130

Bread *(cont.)*

wheat *(Arnold Brick Oven)* 80
wheat *(Arnold Sunny Valley)*, 2 slices 100
wheat *(Pepperidge Farm/Pepperidge Farm Natural)* 90
wheat *(Pepperidge Farm Family)* 70
wheat, cracked, thin *(Pepperidge Farm)* 70
wheat, dark or hearty *(Arnold/Brownberry Bran'nola)* 90
wheat, honey *(Healthy Choice)* 60
wheat, light *(Pepperidge Farm)*, 3 slices 130
wheat, light, golden *(Arnold)*, 2 slices 80
wheat, sesame, hearty *(Pepperidge Farm)* 100
wheat, very thin *(Pepperidge Farm)*, 3 slices 110
wheat, whole *(Arnold Stoneground 1 lb. 4 oz.)* 60
wheat, whole *(Arnold Stoneground 2 lb.)*, 2 slices 100
wheat, whole *(Wonder 24 oz.)* 80
wheat, whole, soft or thin *(Pepperidge Farm)* 60
wheatberry *(Healthy Choice)* 80
wheatberry, honey *(Arnold)* 70
wheatberry, honey *(Arnold Bran'nola)* 90
wheatberry, honey, hearty *(Pepperidge Farm)* 100
white *(Arnold Brick Oven)* 80
white *(Arnold Brick Oven 1 lb.)*, 2 slices 130
white *(Brownberry Natural)*, 2 slices 120
white *(Wonder 12 oz.)*, 2 slices 100
white *(Wonder 1 lb.)* 60
white, sandwich *(Pepperidge Farm)*, 2 slices 130
white, soft *(Arnold Country/Brownberry)* 80
white, soft *(Brownberry 16 oz.)*, 2 slices 110
white, split top *(Healthy Choice)* 60
white, toasting *(Pepperidge Farm)* 90
white, thin *(Pepperidge Farm)* 80
white, very thin *(Pepperidge Farm)*, 3 slices 110
white or wheat *(Home Pride 20 oz.)* 70
white or wheat *(Wonder Low Fat)*, 2 slices 80
Bread, brown, canned:
(S&W), ½ slice, 1.6 oz. 90
plain or raisin *(B&M)*, ½ slice 130
Bread, frozen, 1 piece:
corn bread, w/1 tbsp. honey butter *(Marie Callender)* . . . 150
garlic *(Marie Callender)* 190

garlic, Parmesan and Romano *(Marie Callender)* 200
Bread, refrigerated:
corn bread twists *(Pillsbury)*, 1 piece 140
French, crusty *(Pillsbury)*, 1/5 loaf 150
Bread crumbs, 1/4 cup, except as noted:
(Contadina), 1/3 cup 100
all varieties *(Devonsheer/Old London)* 100
garlic and herb, lemon herb, or Parmesan *(Progresso)* . 100
plain or Italian style *(Progresso)* 110
tomato basil *(Progresso)* 120
Bread cubes, see "Stuffing"
Bread mix*, 1/6 loaf, except as noted:
corn bread *(Ballard)*, 1/18 loaf 130
corn bread, buttermilk *(Martha White)*, 1/5 loaf 150
corn bread, chili fiesta *(Martha White)* 190
corn bread, golden honey *(Martha White)* 170
corn bread, Mexican *(Gladiola)* 130
corn bread, Mexican *(Martha White)* 140
corn bread, yellow *(Martha White)*, 1/5 loaf 140
corn bread, white or yellow *(Gladiola)* 140
wheat or white *(Pillsbury* Bread Machine), 1/12 loaf 130
Bread mix, sweet, 1/12 loaf*:
apple cinnamon or blueberry *(Pillsbury* Quick) 180
banana, nut, or pumpkin *(Pillsbury* Quick) 170
carrot *(Pillsbury* Quick) 140
cinnamon swirl *(Pillsbury* Quick) 220
cranberry *(Pillsbury* Quick) 160
date or lemon poppy seed *(Pillsbury* Quick) 180
Breadfruit nut *(Goya* Pana de Pepita), 4 pieces 40
Breadstick:
(Stella D'Oro), 1 stick 40
all varieties:
    (Stella D'Oro Fat Free Original Deli), 5 sticks 60
    (Stella D'Oro Fat Free Original Grissini), 3 sticks 60
    (Stella D'Oro Fat Free Traditional), 2 sticks 70
cheddar, thin *(Pepperidge Farm)*, 7 sticks 70
cheese, three *(Pepperidge Farm)*, 9 sticks 140
garlic, onion, or wheat *(Stella D'Oro)*, 1 stick 40
onion, thin *(Pepperidge Farm)*, 7 sticks 70
pumpernickel *(Pepperidge Farm)*, 9 sticks 150

Breadstick *(cont.)*

sesame *(Pepperidge Farm)*, 9 sticks 160

sesame *(Stella D'Oro)*, 1 stick 50

Breadstick, refrigerated *(Pillsbury)*, 1 piece 110

Broad beans:

fresh, boiled, drained, 4 oz. 64

dried, boiled, ½ cup 93

dried, canned *(Progresso* Fava Beans), ½ cup 110

Broccoli, fresh:

raw, spear, 8.7 oz. 42

boiled, drained, 1 spear, 6.3 oz. 51

boiled, drained, chopped, ½ cup 22

Broccoli, frozen:

(Seneca), 1 cup 25

spears *(Green Giant)*, 3 oz. 25

florets *(Green Giant)*, 1⅓ cups 25

chopped *(Green Giant)*, ¾ cup 25

chopped *(Seabrook)*, ¾ cup, 3 oz. 25

cuts *(Green Giant)*, 1 cup 25

in butter sauce, spears *(Green Giant)*, 4 oz. 50

in cheese sauce *(Green Giant)*, ⅔ cup 70

Broccoli, cheese-breaded, frozen *(Giorgio)*, 10 pieces,

1.1 oz. 210

Broccoli combinations (see also "Vegetables, mixed"),

frozen:

carrots, cauliflower *(Green Giant American Mixtures)*,

¾ cup 25

carrots, water chestnuts *(Birds Eye)*, ½ cup 30

cauliflower *(Birds Eye)*, ½ cup 20

cauliflower, carrots:

(Birds Eye), ½ cup 25

(Green Giant Harvest Fresh), 1 cup 30

in cheese sauce *(Birds Eye)*, ½ cup 70

in cheese sauce *(Green Giant)*, ⅔ cup 80

corn and peas, in butter sauce *(Green Giant)*,

¾ cup 60

cauliflower, red peppers *(Birds Eye)*, ½ cup 20

corn, red peppers *(Birds Eye)*, ½ cup 50

green beans, onions, red peppers *(Birds Eye)*, ½ cup . . .25

pasta, peas, corn, peppers, in butter sauce *(Green Giant)*, ¾ cup 70
Broccoli rabe *(Frieda's* Rapini), ¾ cup, 3 oz. 15
Broth, see "Bouillon" and "Soup"
Brown gravy, ¼ cup:
w/onions *(Franco-American)* 25
savory *(Heinz)* 25
mix* *(Durkee/French's)* 10
mix*, herb *(Durkee/French's)* 15
Brownie, 1 piece:
chocolate *(Awrey's* Decadent/Sensation) 230
chocolate, Bavarian *(Awrey's)* 250
fudge, w/ or w/out nuts *(Awrey's)* 200
fudge nut *(Awrey's)* 190
fudge nut, chewy *(Awrey's)* 210
fudge walnut *(Tastykake)* 370
Brownie mix*, 1 piece:
(Betty Crocker Original) 180
blonde, w/white chocolate chunks *(Duncan Hines)* 170
caramel or chocolate chunk *(Betty Crocker)* 190
cheesecake swirl *(Pillsbury* Thick 'n Fudgy) 170
chocolate *(Pillsbury* Deluxe) 180
chocolate, double *(Pillsbury* Thick 'n Fudgy) 150
chocolate, German *(Betty Crocker)* 220
chocolate fudge *(Pillsbury* Deluxe 15 oz.) 150
chocolate fudge, dark *(Betty Crocker)* 190
chocolate fudge, hot *(Pillsbury* Deluxe) 160
dark 'n chunky *(Duncan Hines)* 160
devil's food *(SnackWell's)* 140
frosted *(Betty Crocker)* 210
fudge (see also "chocolate fudge," above):
  (Betty Crocker) 190
  (Betty Crocker Family Size) 170
  (Martha White Chewy Family Size) 180
  (Martha White Chewy Snack Size) 160
  (Pillsbury 15 oz.) 150
  (Pillsbury 21.5 oz.) 180
  chewy *(Duncan Hines)* 160
  hot *(Pillsbury)* 160
milk chocolate chunk *(Duncan Hines)* 170

Brownie mix *(cont.)*
Mississippi mud *(Duncan Hines)* 160
peanut butter candies w/*Reese's Pieces (Betty Crocker)* . 200
raspberry dark chocolate *(Duncan Hines)* 150
walnut *(Betty Crocker)* 200
walnut *(Martha White* Deluxe Family Size) 170
walnut *(Pillsbury* Thick 'n Fudgy) 190
Brussels sprouts:
fresh, boiled, drained, 1 sprout, .7 oz. 8
fresh, boiled, drained, ½ cup 30
frozen, boiled, drained, ½ cup 33
frozen, baby, in butter sauce *(Green Giant)*, ⅔ cup 60
Buckwheat flour *(Arrowhead Mills)*, ¼ cup 100
Buckwheat groats:
brown *(Arrowhead Mills)*, ¼ cup 140
roasted, cooked, 1 cup 182
Bulgur (see also "Tabouli"):
dry *(Arrowhead Mills)*, ¼ cup 150
cooked, 1 cup 152
Bun, sweet (see also "Danish"), 1 piece:
cinnamon roll *(Awrey's* Homestyle) 270
cinnamon roll *(Hostess)* 210
honey *(Grandma's)* 410
honey *(Morton)*, 2.3 oz. 290
honey *(Morton* Mini), 1.3 oz. 160
honey, glazed *(Hostess)* 320
honey, glazed or iced *(Tastykake)* 350
honey, iced *(Hostess)* 390
Bun, sweet, frozen or refrigerated, 1 piece:
caramel *(Pillsbury)* 170
cinnamon *(Pepperidge Farm)* 250
cinnamon *(Sara Lee* Deluxe) 320
cinnamon or apple cinnamon, iced *(Pillsbury)* 150
cinnamon raisin or orange, iced *(Pillsbury)* 170
Burbot, meat only, baked or broiled, 4 oz. 130
Burdock root, Japanese *(Frieda's* Gobo), ¾ cup, 3 oz. . 60
Burger King, 1 serving:
breakfast:
    biscuit w/bacon, egg, cheese 510
    biscuit w/sausage 590

Croissan'wich, sausage, egg, cheese 600
French toast sticks 500
hash browns 220
A.M. Express jam, grape or strawberry 30
sandwiches:
  BK Big Fish 700
  BK Broiler chicken 550
  cheeseburger, regular 380
  cheeseburger, double 600
  cheeseburger, double, w/bacon 640
  chicken sandwich 710
  Double Whopper 870
  Double Whopper w/cheese 960
  hamburger 330
  Whopper 640
  Whopper w/cheese 730
  Whopper Jr. 420
  Whopper Jr. w/cheese 460
Chicken Tenders, 8 pieces 310
dipping sauces, 1 oz., except as noted:
  A.M. Express 80
  barbecue 35
  Bull's Eye, ½ oz. 20
  honey 90
  ranch 170
  sweet and sour 45
side dishes:
  fries, medium 370
  fries, coated, medium 340
  onion rings 310
salad, w/out dressing:
  chicken, broiled 200
  garden 100
  side 60
salad dressings, 1.1 oz.:
  bleu cheese 160
  French or Thousand Island 140
  Italian, reduced-calorie light 15
  ranch 180

Burger King (cont.)

desserts and shakes:

Dutch apple pie	300
shake, chocolate, medium	320
shake, chocolate w/syrup, medium	440
shake, strawberry w/syrup, medium	420
shake, vanilla, medium	300

Burrito, frozen:

bean and cheese *(Old El Paso)*, 5 oz.	300
bean and cheese *(Patio)*, 5 oz.	300
bean and cheese *(Tina's)*, 5 oz.	340
beef *(Tina's* Red Hot), 5 oz.	370
beef and bean, all varieties *(Old El Paso)*, 5 oz.	320
beef and bean, mild *(Patio)*, 5 oz.	330
beef and bean, medium *(Patio)*, 5 oz.	310
beef and bean, hot *(Patio)*, 5 oz.	320
beef steak and bean *(Don Miguel)*, 7 oz.	370
chicken *(Don Miguel)*, 7 oz.	360
chicken *(Patio)*, 5 oz.	290
chili, red *(Hormel Quick Meal)*, 4 oz.	280
pizza, cheese *(Old El Paso)*, 3.5 oz.	240
pizza, pepperoni *(Old El Paso)*, 3.5 oz.	260
pizza, sausage *(Old El Paso)*, 3.5 oz.	250

Burrito, breakfast, frozen, 1 pkg.:

egg, scrambled *(Great Starts* Original)	200
egg, scrambled, and bacon *(Great Starts)*	250
ham and cheese *(Great Starts)*	210
hot and spicy *(Great Starts)*	220
sausage *(Great Starts)*	240

Burrito dinner, frozen:

beef *(Chi-Chi's* Burro), 15 oz.	570
chicken *(Chi-Chi's* Burro), 15 oz.	530
chicken con queso *(Healthy Choice)*, 10.55 oz.	350
Burrito dinner mix *(Old El Paso)*, 1 piece*	280

Burrito seasoning mix:

(Lawry's), 1 tbsp.	35
(Old El Paso), 2 tsp.	15

Butter, salted or unsalted, 1 tbsp.:

(Land O Lakes)	100
light *(Land O Lakes)*	50

whipped *(Land O Lakes)* 70
Butter, clarified *(Purity Farms Ghee)*, 1 tsp. 45
Butter, flavored, 1 tbsp.:
garlic flavored *(Land O Lakes)* 100
honey flavored *(Land O Lakes)* 90
Butter beans, see "Lima beans"
Butterbur, canned, chopped, ½ cup 2
Buttercup squash *(Frieda's)*, ¾ cup, 3 oz. 30
Butterfish, meat only, baked, broiled, or microwaved,
    4 oz. 212
Buttermilk, see "Milk"
Butternut squash:
(Frieda's), ¾ cup, 3 oz. 40
fresh, baked, cubed, ½ cup 41
Butterscotch topping, 2 tbsp.:
(Kraft) 130
caramel *(Smucker's* Nonfat/Special Recipe) 130

C

Cabbage, fresh:
raw *(Dole)*, $1/_{12}$ medium head 25
boiled, drained, shredded, $1/_2$ cup 17
bok choy, raw *(Frieda's)*, 1 cup, 3 oz. 10
bok choy, boiled, drained, shredded, $1/_2$ cup 10
Chinese, raw, shredded *(Dole)*, $1/_2$ cup 5
napa, raw *(Dole)*, 3 oz. 6
napa, raw *(Frieda's)*, 1 cup, 3 oz. 10
pe-tsai, raw, shredded, $1/_2$ cup 6
pe-tsai, boiled, drained, shredded, $1/_2$ cup 8
red, raw, shredded *(Dole)*, 3 oz. 25
red, boiled, drained, shredded, $1/_2$ cup 16
savoy, raw, shredded, $1/_2$ cup 10
savoy, boiled, drained, shredded, $1/_2$ cup 18
Cabbage, sweet and sour, red, canned or in jars:
(Greenwood), $1/_2$ cup 100
(S&W), 2 tbsp. 15
(Seneca), $1/_2$ cup 80
Cactus leaves or pads *(Frieda's)*, $3/_4$ cup, 3 oz. 20
Cactus pear, see "Prickly pear"
Cake, $1/_{16}$ cake, except as noted:
banana *(Awrey's Sheet)*, $1/_{24}$ cake 350
banana chocolate chip *(Awrey's Marquise)* 310
Black Forest torte *(Awrey's)*, $1/_{12}$ cake 350
Boston creme *(Awrey's)* 190
carrot, cream cheese iced *(Awrey's)* 390
carrot supreme *(Awrey's Sheet)*, $1/_{24}$ cake 400
cherries cordial *(Awrey's Marquise)* 240
chocolate:
   double *(Awrey's Sheet)*, $1/_{24}$ cake 310
   double *(Awrey's Torte)*, $1/_{12}$ cake 340
   double, 2 layer *(Awrey's)* 250
   German *(Awrey's Sheet)*, $1/_{24}$ cake 340

Cake, chocolate *(cont.)*

German, layer *(Awrey's)* 360
peanut *(Awrey's* Marquise) 330
tropical *(Awrey's* Marquise) 230
white iced, layer *(Awrey's)* 270
coconut buttercream *(Awrey's* Sheet), ¹/₂₄ cake 380
coconut buttercream, layer *(Awrey's)* 360
coffee cake *(Awrey's* Long John), ¹/₁₂ cake 190
espresso, French *(Awrey's* Marquise) 320
fruit *(Hostess)*, ¹/₁₂ cake 510
lemon layer *(Awrey's)* 320
Neapolitan *(Awrey's)*, ¹/₁₂ cake 360
orange, frosty *(Awrey's* Sheet), ¹/₂₄ cake 350
orange, layer *(Awrey's)* 330
peach, Georgia *(Awrey's* Marquise) 260
pound, golden *(Awrey's)*, ¹/₆ cake 250
raspberry and creme *(Awrey's* Marquise) 260
raspberry nut *(Awrey's* Marquise) 310
sponge, uniced *(Awrey's)*, ¹/₂₄ cake 190
strawberry supreme *(Awrey's* Marquise) 240
strawberry supreme, torte *(Awrey's)*, ¹/₁₂ cake 270
yellow, lemon iced, 2 layer *(Awrey's)* 290
yellow, white iced *(Awrey's* Sheet), ¹/₂₄ cake 360

Cake, frozen:

Boston creme *(Mrs. Smith's)*, ¹/₈ cake 170
carrot *(Oregon Farms)*, ¹/₆ cake 280
cheesecake *(Sara Lee* Original Cream), ¹/₄ cake 330
chocolate:
double, layer *(Sara Lee)*, ¹/₈ cake 260
fudge *(Amy's)*, 3.25 oz. 320
fudge or German, layer *(Pepperidge Farm)*, ¹/₆ cake . 300
fudge stripe layer *(Pepperidge Farm)*, ¹/₆ cake 290
German *(Sara Lee)*, ¹/₈ cake 280
mousse *(Pepperidge Farm)*, ¹/₈ cake 250
mousse *(Sara Lee)*, ¹/₅ cake 400
raspberry royale *(Weight Watchers)*, 3.5 oz. 190
coconut *(Sara Lee)*, ¹/₈ cake 280
coconut layer *(Pepperidge Farm)*, ¹/₆ cake 300
coffee cake *(Sara Lee)*, ¹/₈ cake 220
coffee cake *(Sara Lee* Reduced Fat), ¹/₆ cake 180

devil's food *(Oregon Farms* Divine), ⅙ cake 260
devil's food, layer *(Pepperidge Farm),* ⅙ cake 290
golden layer *(Pepperidge Farm),* ⅙ cake 290
golden layer, fudge *(Sara Lee),* ⅛ cake 270
lemon mousse *(Pepperidge Farm),* ⅛ cake 250
pineapple cream *(Pepperidge Farm),* ⅑ cake 240
pound:
   (Sara Lee Reduced Fat), ¼ cake 280
   butter *(Pepperidge Farm),* ⅕ cake 290
   butter *(Sara Lee),* ¼ cake 320
   chocolate swirl *(Sara Lee),* ¼ cake 330
   strawberry swirl *(Sara Lee),* ¼ cake 290
strawberry cream *(Pepperidge Farm),* ⅑ cake 230
strawberry stripe layer *(Pepperidge Farm),* ⅙ cake 310
vanilla layer *(Pepperidge Farm),* ⅙ cake 290
Cake, mix*, 1/12 cake, except as noted:
angel food *(Pillsbury Moist Supreme)* 140
angel food *(SuperMoist* Traditional) 130
banana *(Duncan Hines* Supreme) 250
banana or butter recipe *(Pillsbury Moist Supreme)* 260
butter pecan *(SuperMoist)* 250
butter recipe, chocolate *(Pillsbury Moist Supreme)* 270
butter recipe, chocolate *(SuperMoist)* 270
butter recipe, fudge or golden *(Duncan Hines),* 1/10 cake . 320
butter recipe, yellow *(SuperMoist)* 260
butterscotch or caramel *(Duncan Hines)* 250
carrot *(Pillsbury Moist Supreme)* 260
carrot *(SuperMoist),* 1/10 cake 320
cheesecake *(Jell-O* Homestyle), ⅙ cake 360
cheesecake *(Jell-O* Real), ⅙ cake 350
cherry, wild *(Duncan Hines)* 250
cherry chip *(SuperMoist),* 1/10 cake 280
chip, rainbow *(SuperMoist)* 250
chocolate, all varieties *(Pillsbury Moist Supreme)* 250
chocolate, all varieties *(SuperMoist)* 250
chocolate caramel nut *(Pillsbury Bundt),* 1/16 cake 290
chocolate chip *(SuperMoist)* 280
cinnamon *(Pillsbury Streusel Swirl),* 1/16 cake 260
devil's food *(Pillsbury Moist Supreme)* 270
devil's food *(SuperMoist)* 240

Cake, mix *(cont.)*
devil's food or yellow *(SuperMoist Light)*, 1/10 cake 230
fudge, hot *(Pillsbury Bundt)* 350
fudge marble or party swirl *(SuperMoist)* 250
fudge swirl *(Pillsbury Moist Supreme)* 250
Funfetti (Pillsbury Moist Supreme) 240
lemon *(Pillsbury Moist Supreme)*, 1/10 cake 300
lemon *(SuperMoist)* 280
lemon, orange, or strawberry *(Duncan Hines Supreme)* . 250
marble, fudge *(Duncan Hines)* 250
peanut butter chocolate swirl *(SuperMoist)* 240
pineapple, key lime, raspberry, or spice *(Duncan Hines)* . 250
pound *(Betty Crocker)*, 1/8 cake 270
spice *(SuperMoist)* 250
strawberry *(Pillsbury Moist Supreme)* 260
strawberry cream cheese *(Pillsbury Bundt)*, 1/16 cake . . . 300
strawberry swirl *(SuperMoist)*, 1/10 cake 290
vanilla, French *(Duncan Hines)* 250
vanilla, French *(Pillsbury Moist Supreme)*, 1/10 cake 300
vanilla, French *(SuperMoist)* 250
vanilla, golden *(SuperMoist)* 280
white *(Duncan Hines)* 240
white *(Pillsbury Moist Supreme/Plus)*, 1/10 cake 280
white *(SuperMoist)* 230
white *(SuperMoist Light)*, 1/10 cake 210
white *(Sweet Rewards Reduced Fat)* 210
white, Olympic party *(SuperMoist)* 240
white, sour cream *(SuperMoist)*, 1/10 cake 280
white 'n fudge swirl *(Pillsbury Moist Supreme)* 250
yellow *(Duncan Hines)* 250
yellow *(Pillsbury Moist Supreme)* 240
yellow *(SuperMoist)* 250
Cake, snack (see also specific listings), 1 piece, except
as noted:
all fruit varieties *(Health Valley* Healthy Tarts) 150
apple *(Health Valley Bakes)* 70
apple or apricot bar *(Health Valley)* 140
banana *(Little Debbie* Twins) 250
banana *(Tastykake* Creamies) 170
Boston creme *(Drake's)* 170

brownie, fudge filled *(Health Valley)* 110
cheesecake *(Boar's Head* New York), 4 oz. 380
cheesecake bar, all varieties *(Health Valley)* 160
chocolate *(Ding Dongs)*, 2 pieces 360
chocolate *(Funny Bones)*, 2 pieces 300
chocolate *(Ho-Hos)*, 3 pieces 380
chocolate *(Hostess Choco-Diles)* 240
chocolate *(Suzy Q's)*, 2 pieces 450
chocolate *(Yodels)*, 2 pieces 280
chocolate chip *(Little Debbie)* 280
coconut covered *(Sno Balls)*, 2 pieces 350
coffee cake *(Drake's)* 130
crumb *(Hostess)*, 3 pieces 360
cupcake, chocolate *(Hostess)*, 2 pieces 360
cupcake, chocolate *(Tastykake)*, 2 pieces 220
cupcake, chocolate, iced, creme *(Tastykake)*, 2 pieces . 250
cupcake, orange *(Hostess)*, 2 pieces 320
date *(Health Valley Bakes)* 70
date bar *(Health Valley)* 140
golden, creme filled *(Hostess* Dessert Cup) 90
golden, creme filled *(Little Debbie Golden Cremes)* 280
golden, creme filled *(Sunny Doodles)*, 2 pieces 220
golden, creme filled *(Twinkies)*, 1.4 oz. 140
jelly filled *(Tastykake Krimpets)*, 2 pieces 190
jelly filled *(Tastykake Krimpets* Low Fat), 2 pieces 180
lemon filled *(Tastykake Krimpets* Low Fat), 2 pieces . . . 180
peanut butter *(Tastykake Kandy Kakes)*, 3 pieces 280
pound cake *(Awrey's)* 210
pound cake *(Tastykake)* 320
raisin *(Health Valley Bakes)* 70
raisin bar *(Health Valley* Fat Free) 140
stick, dunking *(Little Debbie)* 250
strawberry shortcake *(Little Debbie)* 290
Swiss roll *(Little Debbie)* 320
vanilla *(Little Debbie)* 380
Calves' liver, see "Liver"
Calzone, refrigerated:
cheese *(Stefano's)*, 6-oz. piece 510
pepperoni *(Stefano's)*, 6-oz. piece 520
spinach *(Stefano's)*, 6-oz. piece 440

Candy:

(Baby Ruth), 2.1-oz. bar	280
(Butterfinger), 2.1-oz. bar	280
butterscotch *(Land O Lakes)*, 3 pieces, .6 oz.	70
candy corn *(Heide/Heide Indian)*, 1 oz.	110
caramel *(Pearson Nips)*, 2 pieces	60
caramel, chocolate coated *(Pom Poms)*, 1.58-oz. box	200
caramel, chocolate coated *(Rolo)*, 1.9 oz.	220
caramel, w/cookies *(Twix Singles)*, 2 bars, 2 oz.	280
chocolate, candy coated *(M&M's)*, 1.5 oz.	210
chocolate, candy coated, w/almonds *(M&M's)*, 1.5 oz.	230
chocolate, candy coated, w/peanuts *(M&M's)*, 1.5 oz.	220
chocolate, dark *(Dove)*, 1/4 of 6-oz. bar	230
chocolate, dark *(Ghirardelli)*, 1.5 oz.	210
chocolate, dark, w/almonds *(Ghirardelli)*, 1.5-oz. bar	220

chocolate, milk:

(Dove), 1/4 of 6-oz. bar	230
(Ghirardelli), 1.25-oz. bar	190
(Hershey's), 1.55-oz. bar	230
(Nestlé), 1.45-oz. bar	220
plain or w/almonds *(Hershey's Nuggets)*, 4 pieces	210
plain or w/almonds *(Hershey's Kisses)*, 8 pieces	210
w/almonds *(Ghirardelli)*, 1.5 oz.	230
w/almonds *(Hershey's)*, 1.45-oz. bar	230
w/caramel *(Caramello)*, 1.6-oz. bar	220
cookies and cream *(Ghirardelli)*, 1.3 oz.	190
w/crisps *(Crunch)*, 1.55-oz. bar	230
w/crisps *(Ghirardelli)*, 1.25-oz. bar	180
w/fruit and nuts *(Chunky)*, 1.4-oz. bar	200
w/macadamias *(Ghirardelli)*, 1.25-oz. bar	190
w/peanuts *(Mr. Goodbar)*, 1.75-oz. bar	270
w/pecans *(Ghirardelli)*, 4 pieces, 1.5 oz.	230
wafers *(Ghirardelli)*, 11 pieces, 1.5 oz.	210
chocolate mint *(Ghirardelli)*, 1.5 oz.	220
chocolate mint, cookies and *(Hershey's)*, 1.55-oz. bar	230
chocolate mint wafers *(Ghirardelli)*, 11 pieces, 1.5 oz.	210
coconut, w/chocolate *(Mounds)*, 1.9-oz. bar	250
coffee *(Pearson Nips)*, 2 pieces	60
creme egg *(Milky Way)*, 1.2-oz. piece	190
creme egg *(Snickers)*, 1.2-oz. piece	170

fruit, all flavors *(Skittles* Singles), 2.2-oz. bag 250
fruit, gummed *(Dots),* 2.25-oz. box 220
fruit, gummed *(Gummi Savers),* 1.5 oz. 130
fruit chews, all flavors *(Starburst),* 8 pieces, 1.4 oz. . . . 160
fruit twists *(Starburst* Singles), 2-oz. bag 190
fudge *(Kraft* Fudgies), 5 pieces, 1.4 oz. 180
gum *(Doublemint/Wrigley's Spearmint),* 1 piece 10
gum *(Juicy Fruit),* 1 piece 10
hard *(Brach's Sparklers),* 3 pieces, .6 oz. 70
hard *(Charms),* 2 pieces, .2 oz. 25
hard *(Lifesavers),* 2 pieces 20
honey *(Bit-O-Honey),* 1.7-oz. bar 200
jelled *(Jujyfruits),* 15 pieces, 1.4 oz. 160
jelled, rings *(Chuckles),* 4 pieces, 1.6 oz. 150
jelly beans *(Smucker's),* 24 pieces, 1.4 oz. 150
licorice *(Crows),* 12 pieces, 1.5 oz. 150
licorice, black or cherry *(Nibs),* 22 pieces 140
licorice, black or strawberry *(Twizzlers),* 4 pieces 140
licorice, bridge mix *(Goelitz),* 2 tbsp., 1.4 oz. 150
licorice, candy coated *(Good & Plenty),* 1.4 oz. 130
lollipop *(Tootsie Pop),* .6-oz. pop 60
(Mars), 1.76-oz. bar 240
marshmallow *(Funmallows),* 4 pieces 110
marshmallow *(Kraft* Jet-Puffed), 5 pieces, 1.2 oz. 110
marshmallow, mini *(Funmallows),* ½ cup 100
(Milky Way Original Singles), 2-oz. bar 270
(Milky Way Dark Singles), 1.76-oz. bar 220
mint, butter *(Kraft),* 7 pieces 60
mint, chocolate coated *(After Eight),* 5 pieces 190
mint, chocolate coated *(Junior Mints),* 1.6-oz. box 180
mint, chocolate coated *(York* Peppermint Pattie), 1.5 oz. . 150
mint, party *(Kraft),* 7 pieces 60
nonpareils *(Sno-Caps),* ¼ cup, 1.4 oz. 190
nougat *(Brach's),* 4 pieces 170
nougat *(Charleston Chew* Vanilla), 5 pieces, 1.2 oz. 150
nougat bar, chocolate coated *(Charleston Chew),* 1.9 oz. . 230
(Oh Henry!), 1.8-oz. bar 230
(100 Grand), 1.5-oz. bar 200
(Pay Day), 1.85-oz. bar 250
peanut *(Planters),* 1.6-oz. bar 230

Candy *(cont.)*

peanut, chocolate coated *(Goobers)*, 1.38 oz. 210
peanut brittle *(Kraft)*, 1.3 oz. 170
peanut butter, candy coated *(Reese's Pieces)*, 1.6-oz.
    bag 230
peanut butter, w/cookie *(Twix)*, .9-oz. bar 130
peanut butter bar *(5th Avenue)*, 2 oz. 280
peanut butter cup *(Reese's)*, 2 pieces, 1.6 oz. 240
pretzel, chocolate coated *(Price's)*, 2 pieces 180
raisins, chocolate coated *(Raisinets)*, 1.58 oz. 200
rock candy *(Brach's)*, 1 oz. 110
(Snickers Singles), 2.07-oz. bar 280
(Snickers Munch), 1.4-oz. bar 230
(Sugar Babies Pouch), 1.7-oz. bag 190
(Sugar Daddy Nuggets), 5 pieces, 1.5 oz. 170
(3 Musketeers), 2.13-oz. bar 260
toffee *(Brach's* Treasures), 3 pieces 80
toffee bar *(Heath)*, 1.4 oz. 210
toffee bar *(Skor)*, 1.4 oz. 220
(Tootsie Roll Midges), 6 pieces, 1.4 oz. 160
wafer, chocolate coated *(Kit Kat)*, 1½-oz. bar 220
(Whatchamacallit), 1.7-oz. bar 250
Cantaloupe, ½ of 5 -diam. melon 94
Cantaloupe cocktail drink *(Snapple)*, 8 fl. oz. 120
Capers:
(Progresso), 1 tsp. 0
w/pimientos *(Goya)*, ¼ cup 25
Cappuccino, iced:
(Jamaican Gold), 11 oz. 145
coffee *(Maxwell House)*, 8 fl. oz. 130
mocha or vanilla *(Maxwell House)*, 8 fl. oz. 140
Cappuccino bar, frozen, see "Ice bar"
Carambola:
fresh *(Frieda's* Starfruit), 5 oz. 45
dried *(Frieda's* Starfruit), ⅓ cup, 1.4 oz. 120
Caramel dip *(Marie's)*, 2 tbsp. 150
Caramel topping, 2 tbsp.:
(Smucker's Sundae/Microwave Fat Free) 110
hot *(Smucker's)* 120
peanut butter *(Smucker's)* 150

Caraway seeds, 1 tsp. 7
Cardamom *(McCormick),* ¼ tsp. 4
Cardoon, boiled, drained, 4 oz. 25
Carnival squash *(Frieda's),* ¾ cup, 3 oz. 30
Carp, meat only, baked or broiled, 4 oz. 184
Carrot:
fresh, raw *(Dole),* 7" long, 1¼" diam., 2.8 oz. 35
fresh, raw, shredded, ½ cup 24
fresh, boiled, drained, sliced, ½ cup 35
canned, all varieties *(Seneca),* ½ cup 25
canned, whole, baby *(LeSueur),* ½ cup 35
canned, whole or sliced *(Stokely),* 4.5 oz. 30
canned, sliced *(Allens/Crest Top),* ½ cup 35
canned, sliced *(Del Monte),* ½ cup 35
canned, sliced *(Green Giant),* ½ cup 25
frozen *(Seneca),* ¾ cup 25
frozen, baby, whole *(Stilwell),* ⅔ cup 35
frozen, baby, cut *(Green Giant),* ¾ cup 30
frozen, crinkle *(Stilwell),* ⅔ cup 35
Carrot juice, 8 fl. oz.:
citrus or tropical *(V-8 Splash)* 120
strawberry-kiwi *(V-8 Splash)* 110
Casaba, ¹⁄₁₀ of 7¾" melon 43
Cashew:
dry- or oil-roasted, 1 oz. or 18 medium 163
oil-roasted *(Planters),* 1-oz. pkg. 160
oil-roasted *(Planters* Fancy), 1 oz. 170
honey-roasted *(Planters),* 1 oz. 150
Catfish, channel, meat only:
farmed, baked or broiled, 4 oz. 172
wild, baked or broiled, 4 oz. 119
Cauliflower:
fresh, raw, 3 flowerets 14
fresh, boiled, drained, 1" pieces, ½ cup 14
fresh, green, raw, ⅕ head 28
fresh, green, boiled, drained, 1" pieces, ½ cup 20
frozen *(Seneca),* 1 cup 20
frozen, florets *(Green Giant),* 1 cup 25
frozen, in cheese sauce *(Green Giant),* ½ cup 60

Caviar (see also "Roe"):
black or red, 1 tbsp. 40
lumpfish, black or red *(Romanoff)*, 1 tbsp. 15
salmon, red *(Romanoff)*, 1 tbsp. 35
Caviar spread *(Krinos* Taramosalata), 1 tbsp. 90
Celeriac, fresh *(Frieda's* Celery Root), ¾ cup, 3 oz. 35
Celery:
fresh *(Dole)*, 2 medium stalks, 3.9 oz. 20
frozen *(Seneca)*, ¾ cup 10
Celery seeds, 1 tsp. 8
Cereal, ready-to-eat (see also specific grains):
almond crunch w/raisins *(Healthy Choice)*, 1 cup 210
amaranth flakes *(Health Valley* Organic), ¾ cup 100
bran *(Kellogg's* Complete), ¾ cup 90
bran *(Kellogg's* All-Bran), ½ cup 80
bran *(Kellogg's* Bran Buds), ⅓ cup 80
bran *(Kellogg's* Frosted Bran), ¾ cup 100
bran *(Nabisco 100% Bran)*, ⅓ cup 80
bran, w/apples and cinnamon *(Health Valley)*, ¾ cup . . . 160
bran, raisin *(Kellogg's)*, 1 cup 200
bran, raisin *(Post)*, 1 cup 190
bran, w/raisins *(Health Valley* Organic), ¾ cup 160
bran, w/raisins *(Total)*, 1 cup 180
bran flakes, raisin *(Health Valley)*, 1¼ cups 190
corn *(Corn Chex)*, 1 cup 110
corn *(Kellogg's Corn Pops)*, 1 cup 120
corn *(Post Toasties)*, 1 cup 100
corn bran *(Quaker* Crunchy), ¾ cup 90
corn and rice *(Kellogg's Crispix)*, 1 cup 110
cornflakes *(Country* Corn Flakes), 1 cup 120
cornflakes *(Kellogg's Corn Flakes)*, 1 cup 100
cornflakes, blue *(Health Valley* Organic), ¾ cup 100
cornflakes, frosted *(Kellogg's Frosted Flakes)*, ¾ cup . . . 120
granola *(C.W. Post* Hearty), ⅔ cup 280
granola *(Heartland)*, ½ cup 300
granola *(Heartland* Low Fat), ½ cup 210
granola *(New Morning Oatiola)*, ¾ cup 200
granola, all varieties *(Health Valley* 98% Fat Free),
⅔ cup 180
granola, w/raisins *(Heartland)*, ½ cup 290

(Healthy Choice Toasted Brown Sugar Squares), 1 cup . 190
kamut *(New Morning Kamutios)*, 1 cup 120
mixed grain *(Cheerios)*, 1 cup 110
mixed grain *(Fiber One)*, ¹/₂ cup 60
mixed grain *(Golden Grahams)*, ³/₄ cup 120
mixed grain *(Grape-Nuts)*, ¹/₂ cup 200
mixed grain *(Grape-Nuts* Flakes), ³/₄ cup 100
mixed grain *(Healthy Choice)*, ³/₄ cup 110
mixed grain *(Just Right* Crunchy Nuggets), 1 cup 210
mixed grain *(Kellogg's Mueslix Golden Crunch)*, ³/₄ cup . 200
mixed grain *(Kix)*, 1¹/₃ cups 120
mixed grain *(Product 19)*, 1 cup 100
mixed grain *(Team* Flakes), 1¹/₄ cups 220
mixed grain *(Total* Whole Grain), ³/₄ cup 110
mixed grain, all varieties *(Granola O's)*, ³/₄ cup 120
mixed grain, bran *(Multi-Bran Chex)*, 1 cup 200
mixed grain, fruit-nut *(Fruit & Fibre)*, 1 cup 210
mixed grain, fruit-nut *(Just Right)*, 1 cup 210
oat *(Cheerios)*, 1 cup 110
oat *(Kellogg's Nut & Honey Crunch)*, 1¹/₄ cups 120
oat *(Kolln* Muesli), ³/₄ cup 200
oat *(Toasty O's*/Honey & Nut *Toasty O's)*, 1 cup 110
oat, apple cinnamon *(Cheerios)*, ³/₄ cup 120
oat, cinnamon *(Quaker Life)*, 1 cup 120
oat, honey graham *(Quaker Oh!s)*, ³/₄ cup 110
oat bran *(Common Sense)*, ³/₄ cup 110
oat bran *(Health Valley* Real), ¹/₂ cup 200
oat bran flakes *(Arrowhead Mills)*, 1 cup 110
oat bran flakes *(Health Valley* Organic), ³/₄ cup 100
rice *(Apple Cinnamon Rice Krispies)*, ³/₄ cup 110
rice *(Rice Krispies)*, 1¹/₄ cups 120
rice *(Special K)*, 1 cup 110
rice, puffed *(Malt-O-Meal)*, 1 cup 60
rice, brown, crisp *(Health Valley)*, 1 cup 110
rice and rye *(Kellogg's Apple Raisin Crisp)*, 1 cup 180
wheat *(Golden Puffs)*, ³/₄ cup 120
wheat *(Honey Frosted Wheaties)*, ³/₄ cup 120
wheat *(Nabisco Frosted Wheat Bites)*, 1 cup 190
wheat *(Nutri-Grain* Golden), ³/₄ cup 100
wheat *(Wheaties)*, 1 cup 110

Cereal, ready-to-eat *(cont.)*
wheat, puffed *(Quaker)*, 1 cup 50
wheat, raisin *(Nutri-Grain* Golden), 1¼ cups 180
wheat, shredded *(Nabisco)*, 2 pieces 160
wheat, shredded *(Nabisco Spoon Size)*, 1 cup 170
Cereal, cooking/hot (see also specific grains), dry:
barley *(Arrowhead Mills Bits O Barley)*, ⅓ cup 140
barley, banana nut *(Fantastic* Cup), 1.6 oz. 170
farina, see "wheat," below
mixed grain *(Roman Meal)*, 1 pkt. 130
mixed grain *(Roman Meal* Instant), 1 pkt. 100
oat bran *(Quaker)*, ½ cup 150
oat flakes, raisin and spice *(H-O* Instant), 1 pkt. 150
oatmeal, instant, 1 pkt., except as noted:
    (H-O), ½ cup 150
    (Maypo), ⅓ cup 150
    (Quaker) 100
    w/apples and cinnamon *(Quaker)* 130
    cinnamon spice *(Quaker)* 170
    maple *(Maypo)*, ½ cup 190
    maple brown sugar *(Quaker)* 160
    raisin, date, and walnut *(Quaker)* 140
    raisin spice *(Quaker)* 160
oats *(H-O* Quick), ½ cup 150
oats *(H-O* Quick Oats'n Fiber), 1 pkt. 110
oats, rolled *(H-O* Instant), 1 pkt. 110
oats, rolled *(Mothers)*, ½ cup 150
oats, rolled *(Quaker* Quick/Old Fashioned), ½ cup 150
oats, toasted *(H-O* Old Fashioned), ⅓ cup 160
rice *(Arrowhead Mills Rice & Shine)*, ¼ cup 150
wheat *(Wheat Hearts)*, ¼ cup 130
wheat *(Wheatena)*, ⅓ cup 150
wheat, all varieties *(Malt-O-Meal)*, 3 tbsp. 120
wheat, whole *(Quaker)*, ½ cup 130
wheat, farina *(H-O)*, 3 tbsp. 120
Chayote, boiled, drained, 1 pieces, ½ cup 19
Cheese (see also "Cheese food" and "Cheese
    product"):
American *(Borden* Loaf/Sharp), 1 oz. 110
American *(Kraft* Deluxe/*Old English)*, 1-oz. slice 110

American *(Land O Lakes)*, 3/4-oz. slice 70
American, light *(Land O Lakes)*, 1 oz. 70
(Bel Paese), medallions, 3/4 oz. 65
blue, crumbled *(Sargento)*, 1 oz., 1/4 cup 100
brick *(Kraft)*, 1 oz. 110
Brie, 1 oz. 95
cheddar *(Alpine Lace* Reduced Fat), 1 oz. 80
cheddar *(Heluva* Good Low Sodium), 1 oz. 110
cheddar *(Kraft Cracker Barrel)*, 1 oz. 110
cheddar *(Land O Lakes/Chedderella)*, 1 oz. 110
cheddar, mild or sharp *(Kraft* 1/3 Less Fat), 1 oz. 80
cheddar, shredded, mild *(Heluva* Good), 1/4 cup 110
Colby *(Alpine Lace* Reduced Fat), 1 oz. 80
Colby *(Land O Lakes)*, 1 oz. 110
Colby, mild *(Heluva* Good Longhorn), 1 oz. 117
Colby jack *(Heluva* Good), 1 oz. 110
Colby jack, shredded *(Heluva* Good), 1/4 cup 110
Colby Monterey Jack *(Kraft)*, 1 oz. 110
cottage, 1/2 cup, except as noted:
    4% *(Sealtest)* 120
    4%, large curd *(Knudsen)* 130
    4%, small curd *(Knudsen)* 120
    2% *(Knudsen)* 100
    2% *(Sealtest)* 90
    1% *(Friendship)* 90
    California style, 4% *(Friendship)* 115
    garden salad, 1% *(Light n' Lively)* 90
    peach, pineapple, or strawberry, 1.5% *(Knudsen)* . . . 110
    peach and pineapple, 1% *(Light n' Lively)* 120
    pineapple or peach, nonfat *(Friendship)* 110
    tropical fruit *(Knudsen)*, 4 oz. 120
cream cheese, 2 tbsp., except as noted:
    (Philadelphia Brand), 1 oz. 100
    (Western Creamy) 70
    chives *(Philadelphia Brand)*, 1 oz. 90
    fat free *(Philadelphia)*, 1 oz. 25
    soft *(Philadelphia Brand)* 100
    soft, light *(Philadelphia Brand)* 70
    soft, chives and onion *(Philadelphia Brand)* 110
    soft, herb and garlic *(Philadelphia Brand)* 110

Cheese, cream cheese *(cont.)*

soft, olive and pimiento *(Philadelphia Brand)* 100
soft, smoked salmon *(Philadelphia Brand)* 100
whipped *(Philadelphia Brand)*, 3 tbsp. 110
curd, extra sharp *(Heluva* Good), 1 oz. 110
Edam *(Boar's Head)*, 1 oz. 90
farmer *(Kraft)*, 1 oz. 100
feta *(Classika* Portions), 1 oz. 100
feta *(Krinos* Imported), 1 oz. 90
fontina *(Classica)*, 1 oz. 110
goat, semisoft type, 1 oz. 103
goat, soft type, 1 oz. 76
Gorgonzola *(Galbani* Dolcelatte), 1 oz. 93
Gouda *(Boar's Head)*, 1 oz. 110
Gouda *(Kraft)*, 1 oz. 110
Gruyère, 1 oz. 117
Havarti *(Boar's Head)*, 1 oz. 110
Havarti *(Kraft Casino)*, 1 oz. 120
hot pepper *(Alpine Lace)*, 1 oz. 80
Jarlsberg *(Sargento)*, 1.2-oz. slice 120
(Laughing Cow Babybel 7 oz.), 1 oz. 100
Limburger *(Kraft Mohawk Valley)*, 1 oz. 90
mascarpone *(Galbani* Imported), 1 oz. 140
Monterey Jack *(Heluva* Good), 1 oz. 100
Monterey Jack *(Land O Lakes)*, 1 oz. 110
Monterey Jack *(Sargento* Sliced), 1 oz. 100
Monterey Jack, shredded *(Heluva* Good), ¼ cup 100
Monterey Jack, jalapeño *(Kraft)*, 1 oz. 110
mozzarella *(Boar's Head)*, 1 oz. 90
mozzarella *(Land O Lakes)*, 1 oz. 80
mozzarella, whole milk *(Heluva* Good), 1 oz. 80
mozzarella, part skim *(Alpine Lace* Reduced Fat), 1 oz. . . 70
mozzarella, part skim, regular, or skim *(Heluva* Good),
    1 oz. 70
mozzarella, shredded *(Heluva* Good), ¼ cup 80
Muenster *(Alpine Lace* Reduced Sodium), 1 oz. 100
Muenster *(Heluva* Good), 1 oz. 100
Muenster *(Sargento* Sliced), 1 oz. 100
Neufchâtel *(Philadelphia Brand)*, 1 oz. 70
Parmesan, grated *(Kraft)*, 2 tsp. 20

Parmesan, grated *(Land O Lakes)*, 1 tbsp. 20
Parmesan, grated *(Sargento)*, 1 tbsp. 25
Parmesan, shredded *(Kraft)*, 2 tsp. 20
Parmesan, shredded *(Sargento)*, ¼ cup 110
Parmesan-Romano, grated *(Sargento)*, 1 tbsp. 25
pimiento, processed *(Kraft* Deluxe), 1 oz. 100
pizza, shredded *(Heluva* Good), ¼ cup 90
Port du Salut, 1 oz. .100
provolone *(Boar's Head)*, 1 oz. 100
provolone *(Sargento* Sliced), 1 oz. 100
ricotta *(Polly-O* Light), ¼ cup 70
ricotta, whole milk *(Polly-O)*, ¼ cup 110
ricotta, part skim *(Polly-O)*, ¼ cup 90
Romano, grated or shredded *(Classica* Pecorino),
    1 tbsp. 20
Roquefort, 1 oz. 105
string *(Polly-O)*, 1 oz. 80
string, snack *(Handi-Snacks/Kraft)*, 1 oz. 80
Swiss *(Alpine Lace* Reduced Fat), 1 oz. 90
Swiss *(Borden)*, 1 oz. 100
Swiss *(Land O Lakes)*, 1 oz. 110
Swiss *(Sargento* Sliced), ¾-oz. slice 80
Swiss, shredded *(Sargento)*, ¼ cup 110
taco, shredded *(Heluva* Good), ¼ cup 110
"Cheese," substitute and nondairy:
(Sandwich-Mate), .7-oz. slice 60
all varieties *(Smart Beat)*, ⅔ oz. 25
all varieties *(Weight Watchers* Fat Free), ¾-oz. slice 30
American *(Cheeztwo/Sandwich-Mate)*, 1 slice 60
American *(Lunchwagon)*, ¾ oz. 70
American, shredded *(Harvest Moon)*, ¼ cup 120
American or Swiss *(Borden)*, 1 slice 60
cheddar *(Borden/Borden* Taco Mate/Fortified), 1 oz. 100
cheddar, shredded *(Sargento)*, ¼ cup 90
Monterey Jack *(Borden)*, 1 oz. 90
mozzarella, shredded *(Borden)*, 1 oz. 90
mozzarella, shredded *(Sargento)*, ¼ cup 80
Cheese dip, 2 tbsp.:
(Chi-Chi's Fiesta) 40
blue *(Kraft* Premium) 45

Cheese dip *(cont.)*
cheddar, jalapeño *(Heluva* Good Light) 30
cheddar, mild *(Frito-Lay)* .50
cheddar, mild *(Old Dutch)* 30
cheddar and mustard *(Heluva* Good Pretzel) 80
chili *(Fritos)* 45
hot *(Price's* Fiesta) 80
jalapeño and cheddar *(Frito-Lay)* 50
nacho *(Frito-Lay)* 45
nacho *(Kraft/Knudsen* Premium) 60
nacho *(Old Dutch)* 35
Parmesan garlic *(Marie's)* 140
salsa *(Heluva* Good Cheese 'N Salsa) 80
salsa *(Tostitos* Con Queso/Con Queso Low Fat) 40
Cheese food (see also "Cheese" and "Cheese spread"):
all varieties *(Kraft* Singles), ¾-oz. slice 70
American *(Heluva* Good), 1 oz. 70
cheddar, sharp or extra sharp *(Cracker Barrel)*, 2 tbsp. . 100
cheddar, port wine, or smoke *(Kaukauna)*, 1 oz. 90
w/garlic or jalapeños *(Kraft)*, 1 oz. 90
jalapeño *(Land O Lakes)*, 1 oz. 90
port wine *(Wispride* Cup), 2 tbsp. 100
shredded *(Velveeta)*, ¼ cup 130
Swiss *(Borden)*, 1 slice 70
Cheese nut log, sharp *(Wispride)*, 2 tbsp. 100
Cheese product (see also "Cheese food"):
(Cheez Whiz Light), 2 tbsp. 80
(Kraft Free Singles), ¾-oz. slice 30
(Velveeta Light), 1 oz. 60
all varieties *(Borden* Fat Free), 1 slice 25
all varieties *(Lite-Line)*, .7-oz. slice 30
American flavor:
   (Alpine Lace), 1 oz. 80
   (Alpine Lace Nonfat), 1 oz. 45
   (Borden Fat Free/Light), ¾-oz. slice 45
   (Borden Lowfat), 1 slice 30
   (Harvest Moon), ⅔ oz. 50
   (Kraft Deluxe 25% Less Fat), ¾-oz. slice 70
   (Kraft Singles Less Fat), ¾-oz. slice 50
   (Light n' Lively 50% Less Fat), ¾-oz. slice 50

cheddar flavor:
   (Alpine Lace Nonfat), 1 oz. 45
   all varieties *(Spreadery)*, 2 tbsp. 80
   sharp *(Kraft* Singles ⅓ Less Fat), ¾-oz. slice 50
   sharp *(Kraft Free* Singles), ¾-oz. slice 30
mozzarella *(Alpine Lace* Nonfat), 1 oz. 45
pimiento *(Spreadery)*, 2 tbsp. 100
Swiss flavor *(Kraft* Singles Less Fat), ¾-oz. slice 50
Swiss flavor *(Kraft Free* Singles), ¾-oz. slice 30
Cheese sauce, 2 tbsp., except as noted:
(Cheez Whiz Squeezable) 100
all varieties *(Kaukauna Micro Melt)* 80
mix *(French's)*, ¼ pkg. 25
nacho *(Kaukauna)* 80
Cheese spread (see also "Cheese" and "Cheese
   product"):
(Squeez-A-Snak), 2 tbsp. 90
all varieties *(Cheez Whiz)*, 2 tbsp. 90
all varieties *(Easy Cheese)*, 2 tbsp. 100
all varieties *(Heluva* Good), 2 tbsp. 90
all varieties *(Velveeta)*, 1 oz. 80
American *(Borden)*, 1 oz. 80
w/bacon *(Kraft)*, 2 tbsp. 90
blue cheese *(Kraft Roka)*, 2 tbsp. 80
w/jalapeños *(Kraft)*, 1 oz. 80
Limburger *(Mohawk Valley)*, 2 tbsp. 80
Neufchâtel, garlic herb or ranch *(Spreadery)*, 2 tbsp. 80
Neufchâtel, vegetable *(Spreadery)*, 2 tbsp. 70
olive and pimiento *(Kraft)*, 2 tbsp. 70
pimiento *(Price's)*, 2 tbsp. 80
pimiento *(Price's* Light), 2 tbsp. 60
sharp *(Old English)*, 2 tbsp. 90
Cheese sticks, mozzarella, breaded, frozen *(Giorgio)*,
   2 pieces 110
Cheeseburger, see "Beef sandwich"
Cherry:
fresh, sour, red, w/pits, ½ cup 26
fresh, sweet, w/pits, ½ cup 52
canned, in heavy syrup, except as noted, ½ cup:
   dark, pitted *(Del Monte)* 100

Cherry, canned *(cont.)*
  red, in water *(Lucky Leaf/Musselman's)* 60
  red *(Comstock/Wilderness)* 140
  sweet, w/pits, dark *(Oregon)* 100
  sweet, pitted, bing or royal Anne *(Oregon)* 110
  sweet, pitted, dark *(S&W)* 140
  sweet, pitted, royal Anne *(Comstock)* 110
  sweet, pitted, royal Anne *(S&W)* 140
frozen, tart, red *(Stilwell)*, 1 cup 60
Cherry, candied *(S&W* Glace), 5 pieces 80
Cherry, dried, pitted:
bing *(Frieda's)*, 1/4 cup, 1.4 oz. 120
tart *(Frieda's)*, 1/3 cup, 1.4 oz. 150
Cherry, maraschino *(S&W)*, 1 piece 10
Cherry drink:
(After the Fall Very Cherry), 8 fl. oz. 100
wild *(Capri Sun)*, 6.75 fl. oz. 110
mix* *(Kool Aid)*, 8 fl. oz. 100
Cherry juice:
(Dole Mountain), 10 fl. oz. 150
(Juicy Juice), 8 fl. oz. 130
(Minute Maid Box), 8.45 oz. 130
Cherry juice blends, 8 fl. oz.:
(Dole Mountain) 120
(Veryfine Juice-Ups) 150
Cherry pocket *(Tastykake)*, 1 piece 370
Chervil, dried *(McCormick)*, 1/4 tsp. . . . . <1
Chestnut, Chinese, shelled, dried, 1 oz. 103
Chestnut, European:
dried, peeled, 1 oz. 105
roasted, peeled, 1 cup or 17 kernels 350
Chicken (see also "Chicken, refrigerated or frozen"):
broiler-fryer, roasted:
  w/skin, 1/2 chicken, 10.5 oz. (15.8 oz. w/bone) 715
  w/skin, 4 oz. 271
  meat only, 4 oz. 215
  meat only, chopped or diced, 1 cup 266
  skin only, 1 oz. 129
  dark meat only, 4 oz. 232
  light meat only, 4 oz. 196

breast, w/skin, ½ breast, 3.5 oz. (8.5 oz. w/bone) . . . 193
drumstick, w/skin, 1.8 oz. (2.9 oz. w/bone) 112
leg, w/skin, 4 oz. (5.7 oz. w/bone) 265
thigh, w/skin, 2.2 oz. (2.9 oz. w/bone) 153
wing, w/skin, 1.2 oz. (2.3 oz. w/bone) 99
capon, roasted, w/skin, ½ capon, 1.4 lb. (2 lb. w/bone) 1,457
capon, roasted, w/skin, 4 oz. 260
Cornish hen, see "Cornish hen"
roaster, roasted, w/skin, ½ chicken, 1 lb. (1.5 lb.
w/bone) 1,071
roaster, roasted, w/skin, 4 oz. 253
stewing, stewed, meat only, chopped or diced, 1 cup . . . 332
Chicken, canned, chunk:
(Hormel), 2 oz. 70
breast *(Hormel/Hormel* No Salt), 2 oz. 60
white *(Swanson* Premium), 3 oz. 80
white, in water *(Swanson* Premium), ¼ cup 60
Chicken, ground:
cooked *(Perdue),* 3 oz. 170
cooked *(Perdue* Burgers), 3 oz. 160
Chicken, refrigerated or frozen (see also "Chicken
entree, frozen"):
whole, cooked:
dark meat *(Perdue/Perdue Oven Stuffer),* 3 oz. 210
dark meat, seasoned *(Perdue),* 4 oz. 260
dark meat, seasoned, roasted *(Perdue),* 4 oz. 190
white meat *(Perdue/Perdue Oven Stuffer),* 3 oz. 170
white meat, cut up *(Perdue),* 3 oz. 160
white meat, cut up *(Perdue* Country), 3 oz. 170
white meat, seasoned, roasted *(Perdue),* 4 oz. 160
barbecued *(Empire* Kosher), 5 oz. edible 280
breast, cooked:
whole *(Perdue),* 3 oz. 160
whole *(Perdue Oven Stuffer),* 3 oz. 150
split, skinless *(Perdue),* 5.8 oz. 240
split, roasted *(Tyson),* ½ breast 250
quarters *(Perdue),* 3 oz. 170
boneless *(Perdue/Perdue Oven Stuffer),* 3 oz. 120
boneless *(Perdue Fit 'n Easy),* 3 oz. 110
boneless, tenderloin *(Perdue),* 3 oz. 100

Chicken, refrigerated or frozen, breast, cooked *(cont.)*

boneless, thin sliced *(Perdue Fit 'n Easy)*, 2 oz. 80
roundelet *(Tyson)*, 2.6-oz. piece 170
skinless, roasted *(Perdue)*, 5.8-oz. piece 240
tenders *(Banquet Fat Free)*, 3 pieces, 3.5 oz. 120
tenders *(Banquet Original)*, 3 pieces, 3.5 oz. 240
tenders, Southern *(Banquet)*, 3 pieces, 3.5 oz. 260

breast, breaded, cooked:
cutlet *(Perdue Original)*, 3.5 oz. 240
cutlet, Parmesan *(Perdue Kit)*, 3 oz. 230
patties *(Perdue Individually Frozen)*, 3 oz. 220
tenderloin *(Perdue)*, 3 oz. 170
tenderloin *(Perdue Individually Frozen)*, 3 oz. 200

breast, seasoned, cooked:
barbecue *(Perdue)*, 3 oz. 130
barbecue or teriyaki *(Perdue Individually Frozen)*,
　4.3 oz. 160
w/barbecue sauce *(Perdue)*, ½ cup 200
Italian *(Perdue Individually Frozen)*, 4.3 oz. 150
Italian or Oriental *(Perdue)*, 3 oz. 100
lemon pepper *(Perdue)*, 3 oz. 90
lemon pepper *(Perdue Individually Frozen)*, 4.3 oz. . 150

chunks *(Country Skillet)*, 5 pieces, 3.3 oz. 270
chunks, breaded, Southern *(Banquet)*, 5 pieces, 4.5 oz. . 270
chunks, cooked *(Tyson Chick'n Chunks)*, 6 pieces,
　3 oz. 280

drumstick, cooked:
(Perdue Individually Frozen), 2.6 oz. 120
roasted *(Perdue)*, 2.2-oz. piece 110
roasted *(Perdue Oven Stuffer)*, 3.6 oz. 190
roasted *(Tyson)*, 3 pieces 330

fried, 3 oz., except as noted:
(Banquet Country/Country Skillet) 270
(Banquet Original/Southern) 280
breast *(Banquet Original)*, 1 piece, 5.5 oz. 410
drums and thighs or hot 'n spicy *(Banquet)* 260
honey barbecue, skinless *(Banquet)* 120
skinless, regular or lemon pepper *(Banquet)* 210
wings, hot 'n spicy *(Banquet)*, 4 pieces, 4 oz. 260

half, roasted, w/out skin *(Tyson)*, 3 oz. 140

leg, whole, roasted *(Perdue/Perdue* Family), 5.6 oz. 370
leg, whole, roasted *(Perdue* Jumbo), 5.5 oz. 360
leg, quarters, raw *(Tyson),* 4 oz. 290
leg, quarters, cooked *(Perdue/Perdue* Value Pack),
   3 oz. 220
nuggets *(Banquet* Original), 6 pieces, 4.5 oz. 270
nuggets *(Country Skillet),* 10 pieces, 3.3 oz. 280
nuggets, breaded *(Perdue),* 5 pieces 240
nuggets, breaded, and cheese *(Perdue),* 5 pieces 270
nuggets, mozzarella *(Banquet),* 6 pieces, 4.5 oz. 280
patties *(Banquet* Original/*Country Skillet),* 1 patty 190
patties, breast *(Banquet* Fat Free), 1 patty 100
patties, Southern *(Banquet),* 1 patty 170
thigh, cooked:
   boneless, skinless *(Perdue Individually Frozen),*
      3.7 oz. 180
   roasted *(Perdue),* 3.2-oz. piece 240
   roasted *(Tyson),* 3.6-oz. piece 270
   roasted, boneless *(Perdue),* 2 thighs, 3.6 oz. 190
   roasted, boneless *(Perdue Oven Stuffer),* 3.3 oz. . . . 170
   roasted, skinless *(Perdue),* 2.7 oz. 160
   seasoned, fajita *(Perdue),* 2.4 oz. 120
   seasoned, honey mustard *(Perdue),* 2.4 oz. 130
wing, roasted *(Perdue* Wingettes), 3 pieces 210
wing, roasted *(Perdue Oven Stuffer* Drummettes),
   2 pieces 170
wing, roasted *(Perdue Oven Stuffer* Wingettes),
   3 pieces 220
wing, hot and spicy *(Perdue),* 3 oz. 190
"Chicken," vegetarian:
canned:
   diced *(Worthington* Chik), ¼ cup 40
   fried *(Worthington FriChik),* 2 pieces 120
   fried *(Worthington FriChik* Low Fat), 2 pieces 80
   fried, w/gravy *(Loma Linda Chik'n),* 2 pieces 210
   sliced *(Worthington* Chik), 3 slices 70
frozen:
   (Worthington Chik-Stiks), 1 piece 110
   nuggets *(Loma Linda),* 5 pieces 240
   nuggets *(Morningstar Farms),* 4 pieces 160

"Chicken," vegetarian, frozen *(cont.)*
    patties *(Morningstar Farms* Chik), 1 patty 150
    patties *(Worthington Crispy Chik),* 1 patty 170
    roll *(Worthington Chic-Ketts),* 2 slices, ⅜ 120
    roll or sliced *(Worthington),* 2 slices 80
  mix *(Loma Linda* Supreme), ⅓ cup 90

Chicken dinner, frozen:
barbecue, mesquite *(The Budget Gourmet),* 11 oz. 270
barbecue, mesquite *(Healthy Choice),* 10.5 oz. 310
barbecue, w/potato, vegetables *(Tyson* BBQ), 1 pkg. . . . 560
boneless *(Swanson Hungry-Man),* 1 pkg. 630
breaded, country *(Healthy Choice),* 10¼ oz. 350
breast, 11 oz.:
    herbed, w/fettuccine *(The Budget Gourmet)* 260
    honey mustard *(The Budget Gourmet)* 310
    roasted, w/herb gravy *(The Budget Gourmet)* 250
broccoli Alfredo *(Healthy Choice),* 11.5 oz. 300
cacciatore *(Healthy Choice),* 12.5 oz. 270
Cantonese *(Healthy Choice),* 10¾ oz. 280
Dijon *(Healthy Choice),* 11 oz. 270
fingers, and BBQ sauce *(Freezer Queen* Meal), 9 oz. . . . 310
Francesca *(Healthy Choice),* 12.5 oz. 330
fried:
    (Banquet Extra Helping), 18 oz. 910
    (Morton), 9 oz. 420
    country, and gravy *(Marie Callender),* 14 oz. 620
    dark portion *(Swanson),* 1 pkg. 580
    dark portion *(Swanson Hungry-Man),* 1 pkg. 780
    Southern *(Banquet* Extra Helping), 17.5 oz. 750
    white *(Banquet* Extra Helping), 18 oz. 820
    white, mostly *(Swanson Hungry-Man),* 1 pkg. 800
    white portion *(Swanson),* 1 pkg. 630
ginger, Hunan *(Healthy Choice),* 12.6 oz. 380
grilled, in garlic sauce *(Swanson),* 1 pkg. 260
grilled, in mushroom sauce *(Marie Callender),* 14 oz. . . . 480
grilled, Southwestern *(Healthy Choice),* 10.2 oz. 260
grilled patties *(Swanson Hungry-Man),* 1 pkg. 700
herb, country *(Healthy Choice),* 12.15 oz. 310
nuggets *(Freezer Queen* Meal), 6 oz. 320
nuggets *(Morton),* 7 oz. 320

nuggets *(Swanson)*, 1 pkg. 590
parmigiana *(Banquet* Extra Helping), 19 oz. 650
parmigiana *(The Budget Gourmet)*, 11 oz. 280
parmigiana *(Healthy Choice)*, 11.5 oz. 330
parmigiana *(Marie Callender)*, 16 oz. 620
parmigiana *(Swanson)*, 1 pkg. 370
patties *(Freezer Queen* Meal), 7.5 oz. 290
patty, breaded *(Morton)*, 6.75 oz. 280
picante *(Healthy Choice)*, 10.75 oz. 250
roasted *(Healthy Choice)*, 11 oz. 230
roasted, herb *(Swanson)*, 1 pkg. 310
sesame, Shanghai *(Healthy Choice)*, 12 oz. 300
sweet and sour *(Healthy Choice)*, 11 oz. 360
sweet and sour *(Marie Callender)*, 14 oz. 530
teriyaki *(The Budget Gourmet)*, 11 oz. 300
teriyaki *(Healthy Choice)*, 11 oz. 270
Chicken entree, canned:
à la king *(Swanson* Main Dish), 1 cup 320
chow mein *(La Choy/Chun King* Bi-Pack), 1 cup 100
chow mein *(La Choy* Entree), 1 cup 80
and dumplings *(Dinty Moore* Cup), 7½ oz. 190
and dumplings *(Swanson* Main Dish), 1 cup 260
hot and spicy *(Chun King* Bi-Pack), 1 cup 100
w/mushroom *(Hunt's* Homestyle), 1 cup 200
noodles and, see "Noodle entree"
Oriental, w/noodles *(La Choy)*, 1 cup 150
and pasta *(Chef Boyardee* Bowl), 7½ oz. 150
salad *(Swanson* Lunch Kit), 1 cup 300
spicy *(La Choy* Szechwan Bi-Pack), 1 cup 100
stew *(Dinty Moore)*, 1 cup 220
stew *(Dinty Moore* Cup), 7½ oz. 180
sweet and sour *(La Choy/Chun King* Bi-Pack), 1 cup . . . 160
teriyaki *(La Choy* Bi-Pack), 1 cup 110
Chicken entree, frozen:
baked, w/potato, gravy *(Stouffer's* Homestyle), 8⅞ oz. . 270
biryani *(Curry Classics)*, 10 oz. 460
chow mein *(Banquet)*, 9 oz. 210
chow mein *(Stouffer's)*, 10⅝ oz. 260
Cordon Bleu *(Marie Callender)*, 13 oz. 590
and dumplings *(Banquet)*, 10 oz. 270

Chicken entree, frozen *(cont.)*

and dumplings *(Marie Callender)*, 1 cup, 1/2 pkg.	250
and dumplings, country *(Banquet* Family Size), 1 cup	290
escalloped, and noodles *(Stouffer's)*, 10 oz.	450
fettuccine *(Stouffer's* Homestyle), 10.5 oz.	390
fettuccine Alfredo *(Banquet)*, 101/4 oz.	420
fettuccine Alfredo *(Healthy Choice)*, 8.5 oz.	260
fiesta *(Lean Cuisine)*, 8.5 oz.	250
fingers, and barbecue sauce *(Banquet)*, 9 oz.	340
Français *(Tyson)*, 8.9 oz.	260
fried *(Banquet* Original), 9 oz.	470
fried, Southern *(Banquet)*, 83/4 oz.	560
fried, white meat *(Banquet)*, 83/4 oz.	480
garlic, Milano *(Healthy Choice)*, 9.5 oz.	240
glazed, country *(Healthy Choice)*, 8.5 oz.	230
grilled *(Banquet)*, 9.9 oz.	330
grilled, w/mashed potato *(Healthy Choice)*, 8 oz.	180
grilled, Sonoma *(Healthy Choice)*, 9 oz.	230
grilled breast, and rice pilaf *(Marie Callender)*, 113/4 oz.	360
gumbo *(Goya* Asopao de Pollo), 1 pkg.	190
herb roasted, w/mashed potato *(Marie Callender)*, 14 oz.	670
honey mustard *(Healthy Choice)*, 9.5 oz.	270
honey mustard *(Lean Cuisine* Cafe Classics), 8 oz.	270
honey mustard *(Smart Ones)*, 8.5 oz.	200
imperial *(Healthy Choice)*, 9 oz.	240
Italian, w/fettuccine *(Lean Cuisine)*, 9 oz.	270
Kiev *(Tyson)*, 9.1 oz.	440
mandarin *(Healthy Choice)*, 10 oz.	280
Marsala *(Marie Callender)*, 14 oz.	450
Mirabella *(Smart Ones)*, 9.2 oz.	170
Monterey *(Stouffer's* Homestyle), 93/8 oz.	410
w/mushroom sauce *(Tyson)*, 8.9 oz.	220
and noodle casserole *(Swanson* Lunch and More), 1 pkg.	300
and noodles *(Marie Callender)*, 13 oz.	520
à l'orange *(Lean Cuisine)*, 9 oz.	250
Oriental style *(Banquet)*, 9 oz.	260
Parmesan *(Lean Cuisine* Cafe Classics), 107/8 oz.	240
parmigiana *(Banquet)*, 9.5 oz.	320

parmigiana *(Stouffer's* Homestyle), 12 oz. 460
parmigiana, w/tomato sauce *(Banquet)*, 1 patty w/sauce . 240
pasta fiesta *(Marie Callender)*, 12.5 oz. 640
pasta primavera *(Banquet)*, 9.5 oz. 320
patty strips, breaded *(Swanson* Lunch and More),
  1 pkg. 340
in peanut sauce *(Lean Cuisine)*, 9 oz. 280
penne pollo *(Weight Watchers)*, 10 oz. 290
piccata *(Lean Cuisine* Cafe Classics), 9 oz. 270
pie *(Banquet)*, 7-oz. pie 380
pie *(Banquet* Hearty), 1 cup, 1/3 pie 480
pie *(Lean Cuisine)*, 9.5 oz. 310
pie *(Marie Callender)*, 9.5-oz. pie 600
pie *(Stouffer's)*, 10-oz. pie 560
pie *(Swanson)*, 1 pkg. 410
pie *(Swanson* Lunch and More Casserole), 1 pkg. 470
pie *(Swanson* Hungry-Man), 1 pkg. 650
pie, au gratin *(Marie Callender)*, 9.5-oz. pie 690
pie, and broccoli *(Banquet)*, 7-oz. pie 380
pie, and broccoli *(Marie Callender)*, 9.5-oz. pie 670
and rice stir-fry casserole *(Swanson* Lunch and More),
  1 pkg. 240
roasted, herb *(Lean Cuisine* Cafe Classics), 8 oz. 210
roasted, herb *(Tyson)*, 11.35 oz. 290
sesame *(Healthy Choice)*, 9.75 oz. 250
sweet and sour *(The Budget Gourmet)*, 10 oz. 330
tikka *(Curry Classics* Makhanwala), 10 oz. 480
and vegetables *(Lean Cuisine)*, 10.5 oz. 250
and vegetables, Marsala *(Healthy Choice)*, 11.5 oz. 240
wings, barbecue *(Tyson)*, 4 pieces, 3.4 oz. 210
Chicken entree mix, stir-fried *(Skillet Chicken Helper)*,
  1 cup* 270
Chicken gravy, 1/4 cup:
canned *(Franco-American)* 40
canned *(Franco-American* Fat Free) 15
canned, giblet *(Franco-American)* 30
canned, slow-roast *(Franco-American)* 25
mix* *(Durkee)* 20
mix* *(French's)* 25
mix*, roasted *(Knorr)* 30

Chicken lunch meat:
breast, barbecue *(Black Bear)*, 2 oz. 70
breast, browned or mesquite *(Healthy Choice)*, 2 oz. 60
breast, oven roasted:
　(Boar's Head Golden), 2 oz. 50
　(Hebrew National), 2 oz. 45
　(Louis Rich Deluxe), 1-oz. slice 30
　(Louis Rich Deli-Thin), 4 slices, 1.8 oz. 50
　(Oscar Mayer Fat Free), 4 slices, 1.8 oz. 45
breast, skinless *(Healthy Choice)*, 2 oz. 45
breast, smoked *(Boar's Head* Hickory), 2 oz. 60
white meat roll *(Tyson)*, 2 slices, 1.3 oz. 60
Chicken pie, see "Chicken entree, frozen"
Chicken sandwich, frozen, 1 piece:
(Hormel Quick Meal) 340
and broccoli *(Healthy Choice Hearty Handfuls)* 320
and cheddar, w/broccoli *(Hot Pockets)* 300
fajita *(Totino's* Big & Hearty) 270
garlic *(Healthy Choice Hearty Handfuls)* 330
grilled *(Tyson* Microwave) 210
and mushrooms *(Healthy Choice Hearty Handfuls)* 310
pastry *(Mrs. Paterson's Aussie Pie)* 460
Chicken sauce (see also specific listings), ½ cup,
　except as noted:
barbecue flavor *(Hunt's Chicken Sensations)*, 1 tbsp. 35
cacciatore *(Ragú Chicken Tonight)* 80
Caesar *(Lawry's)*, 2 tbsp. 30
country French *(Ragú Chicken Tonight)* 130
creamy, w/mushrooms *(Ragú Chicken Tonight)* 110
creamy, primavera *(Ragú Chicken Tonight)* 90
herbed, w/wine *(Ragú Chicken Tonight)* 80
sherried *(Lawry's)*, 1 tbsp. 20
sweet and sour *(Ragú Chicken Tonight)* 120
Thai, satay *(Lawry's)*, 1 tbsp. 35
wing, Buffalo *(World Harbors* Hot Zings), 1 tbsp. 30
wing, hot *(Nance's)*, 2 tbsp. 15
wing, mild *(Nance's)*, 2 tbsp. 20
Chicken seasoning and coating mix:
(Shake'n Bake Original Recipe), ⅛ pkg. 40
barbecue glaze *(Shake'n Bake)*, ⅛ pkg. 45

coq au vin *(Knorr* Recipe), 1 tbsp. 30
Dijonne *(Knorr* Recipe), ⅙ pkg. 30
extra crispy *(Oven Fry)*, ⅛ pkg. 60
homestyle flour *(Oven Fry)*, ⅛ pkg. 40
hot and spicy *(Shake'n Bake)*, ⅛ pkg. 40
Chicken spread:
chunky *(Underwood)*, ¼ cup 120
salad *(Libby's Spreadables)*, ⅓ cup 140
w/crackers *(Red Devil* Snackers), 1 pkg. 280
Chick-fil-A, 1 serving:
chicken dishes:
  chargrilled, 2.8 oz. 130
  Chick-fil-A Nuggets, 8-pack 290
  Chick-n-Strips, 4 pieces 230
  Chick-n-Strips salad 290
  salad, chargrilled garden 170
  salad plate 290
chicken sandwiches:
  regular or chargrilled deluxe 290
  chargrilled 280
  chargrilled club, w/out dressing 390
  Chick-n-Q 370
  deluxe 300
  salad, whole wheat 320
side dishes, small:
  carrot raisin salad 150
  chicken soup, 1 cup 110
  coleslaw 130
  tossed salad 70
  Waffle fries, salted or unsalted 290
desserts:
  brownie, fudge nut 350
  cheesecake 270
  cheesecake, w/blueberry or strawberry 290
  Icedream, small cone 140
  Icedream, small cup 350
  lemon pie 280
Chickpeas (garbanzos), canned, ½ cup:
(Allens/East Texas Fair) 120
(Eden Organic/Organic Jars) 120

Chickpeas *(cont.)*
(Old El Paso) 100
(Stokely) 110
Chicory, witloof *(Frieda's* Belgium Endive), 2 cups,
  3 oz. 15
Chicory greens, trimmed, 1 oz. 7
Chili, canned, 1 cup, except as noted:
w/beans *(Gebhardt)* 320
w/beans *(Libby's)* 420
w/beans *(Old El Paso)* 200
w/beans *(Van Camp's)* 350
w/beans *(Wolf)* 330
w/beans, jalapeño *(Wolf)* 330
w/out beans *(Libby's)* 480
w/out beans *(Wolf)* 420
w/out beans, hot *(Hormel)* 410
w/out beans, jalapeño *(Wolf)* 420
turkey, w/beans *(Hormel)* 220
vegetarian *(Natural Touch)* 170
vegetarian *(Worthington)* 290
vegetarian *(Worthington* Low Fat) 170
vegetarian, all varieties *(Health Valley* Nonfat), ½ cup 80
Chili, frozen:
w/beans *(Stouffer's* Entree), 8¾ oz. 270
and corn bread *(Marie Callender),* 1 cup,
  1½ corn bread 350
vegetarian *(Tabatchnik* Side Dish), 7.5 oz. 210
Chili, mix, 4 bean *(Knorr* Cup), 1 pkg. 230
Chili base, canned *(Hunt's* Homestyle Fixings), ½ cup . . 85
Chili beans (see also "Mexican beans"), canned,
  ½ cup:
(Gebhardt) 135
(Hunt's) 85
(S&W) 110
hot *(S&W* Chipotle) 90
w/jalapeños and red peppers *(Eden* Organic) 130
spicy *(Green Giant/Joan of Arc)* 110
in zesty sauce *(Campbell's)* 130
Chili pepper, see "Pepper, chili"
Chili powder, 1 tbsp. 24

Chili sauce (see also "Pepper sauce"):
(Del Monte), 1 tbsp. 20
(Hunt's), 2 tsp. 35
(Las Palmas), ¼ cup 15
(Nance's), 2 tbsp. 25
(S&W Steakhouse), 1 tbsp. 15
hot dog *(Gebhardt)*, ¼ cup 60
hot dog *(Wolf)*, 1 tbsp. 15
hot dog, w/beef *(Stenger)*, ¼ cup 70
Chili seasoning mix:
(Durkee Pot-O), ⅛ pkg. 30
(Gebhardt Chili Quick), 2 tbsp. 40
(Lawry's Tex-Mex), 2 tbsp. 50
(Mick Fowler's 2-Alarm Kit), 3 tbsp. 60
(Old El Paso), 1 tbsp. 25
regular or mild *(Durkee)*, ⅕ pkg. 30
Texas red *(Durkee)*, ⅓ pkg. 45
Chimichanga, frozen:
beef *(Old El Paso)*, 1 piece* 360
beefsteak and bean *(Don Miguel)*, 7 oz. 410
chicken *(Don Miguel)*, 7 oz. 400
chicken *(Old El Paso)*, 1 piece* 340
Chimichanga entree, frozen *(Banquet)*, 9.5 oz. 500
Chives, fresh or freeze-dried, chopped, 1 tbsp. 1
Chives, Asian *(Frieda's* Gil Choy), 1 tbsp. 0
Chocolate, see "Candy"
Chocolate, baking:
bar, bittersweet or semisweet *(Hershey's)*, ½ oz. 80
bar, milk *(Ghirardelli)*, 3 squares, 1.5 oz. 220
bar, semisweet *(Baker's)*, 1 oz. 130
bar, white *(Baker's)*, 1 oz. 160
chips or morsels, all varieties *(Hershey's)*, ½ oz.,
　1 tbsp. 80
chips or morsels, milk *(Baker's)*, ½ oz., 1 tbsp. 70
chunks *(Hershey's* Semisweet), 6 chunks 80
kisses *(Hershey's* Mini), 11 pieces 80
semisweet *(M&M's)*, ½ oz. 70
Chocolate drink *(Yoo-Hoo)*, 9 fl. oz. 150
Chocolate milk, chilled, 1 cup:
(Nestlé Quik) 230

Chocolate milk *(cont.)*
low-fat *(Hershey's)* 190
low-fat *(Nestlé Quik)* 190
fat free *(Hershey's)* 130
Chocolate shake *(Nestlé Quik)*, 9 fl. oz. 300
Chocolate syrup, 2 tbsp.:
(Fox's U-Bet) 120
(Smucker's Sundae) 110
(Smucker's Guilt Free) 100
Chocolate topping, 2 tbsp.:
all varieties *(Smucker's Magic Shell)* 220
caramel *(Hershey's)* 100
cherry Melba *(Dickinson's Black Forest)* 130
dark *(Dove)* 140
double *(Hershey's)* 110
fudge *(Smucker's)* 130
fudge *(Smucker's Microwave)* 130
fudge, light *(Smucker's)* 90
fudge, double *(Hershey's)* 120
fudge, hot *(Hershey's)* 130
fudge, hot *(Smucker's/Smucker's Special Recipe)* 140
fudge, hot *(Smucker's Microwave)* 130
fudge, hot *(Smucker's Microwave Fat Free)* 110
fudge, hot *(Smucker's Guilt Free)* 100
milk *(Dove)* 130
mint *(Hershey's)* 110
Chowchow *(Crosse & Blackwell)*, 1 tbsp. 10
Church's Chicken, 1 serving:
chicken, edible portion:
  breast, 2.8 oz. 200
  leg, 2 oz. 140
  Tender Strip, 1.1 oz. 80
  thigh, 2.8 oz. 230
  wing, 3.1 oz. 250
sides:
  biscuit 250
  Cajun rice 130
  coleslaw 92
  corn on cob 139
  fries 210

okra 210
potatoes and gravy 90
apple pie 280
Chutney, mango *(Patak's* Major Grey's), 1 tbsp. 50
Cilantro, see "Coriander"
Cinnamon, ground, 1 tsp. 6
Citron, candied *(S&W),* 39 pieces, 1.1 oz. 90
Citrus drink, 8 fl. oz.:
(Five Alive) 120
punch *(Minute Maid)* 120
punch *(Tropicana)* 140
punch, tropical *(Five Alive)* 110
Citrus salad, in jars, in light syrup *(Sunfresh),* ½ cup . . 70
Clam, meat only:
raw, 9 large or 20 small, 6.3 oz. 133
boiled, poached, or steamed, 4 oz. 168
Clam, canned, ¼ cup or 2 oz.:
chopped or minced *(Doxsee)* 25
minced *(Progresso)* 25
smoked *(S&W)* 130
Clam, fried, frozen:
(Gorton's Crunchy), 3 oz. 260
(Mrs. Paul's), 28 pieces, 3 oz. 280
Clam dip, 2 tbsp.:
(Breakstone's Chesapeake) 50
(Heluva Good New England) 50
(Nalley) 100
Clam juice *(S&W),* 9.6 fl. oz. 20
Clam sauce, canned, ½ cup:
red *(Progresso)* 80
white *(Progresso)* 130
white *(Progresso* Authentic) 90
white, creamy *(Progresso)* 110
Cloves, ground, 1 tsp. 7
Cobbler, frozen:
apple *(Marie Callender),* ¼ pkg. 350
apple or apricot *(Stilwell),* ⅛ pkg. 240
berry or cherry *(Marie Callender),* ¼ pkg. 390
berry, cherry, or blackberry *(Stilwell),* ⅛ pkg. 250
blackberry *(Stilwell),* ⅛ pkg. 250

Cobbler *(cont.)*
blueberry *(Marie Callender)*, ¼ pkg. 340
blueberry *(Pet-Ritz)*, ⅙ pkg. 280
peach *(Marie Callender)*, ¼ pkg. 370
peach *(Stilwell)*, ⅛ pkg. 240
strawberry *(Stilwell)*, ⅛ pkg. 260
Cocktail sauce, see "Seafood cocktail sauce"
Cocoa, baking, unsweetened *(Hershey's)*, 1 tbsp. 20
Cocoa mix, chocolate, 1 pkt.:
(Swiss Miss Lite) 75
(Swiss Miss Marshmallow Lovers) 140
all flavors, except light chocolate supreme and
   chocolate–black cherry *(Land O Lakes* Cocoa
   Classics) 160
and cream *(Swiss Miss)* 155
chocolate *(Swiss Miss* Chocolate Sensation) 150
chocolate *(Swiss Miss* Rich) 110
chocolate, milk or w/marshmallows *(Swiss Miss)* 120
chocolate, Suisse truffle *(Swiss Miss* Premiere) 140
chocolate, white *(Swiss Miss)* 110
chocolate almond mocha *(Swiss Miss* Premiere) 145
chocolate–black cherry *(Land O Lakes* Cocoa Classics) . 150
chocolate English toffee *(Swiss Miss* Premiere) 140
chocolate raspberry truffle *(Swiss Miss* Premiere) 145
chocolate supreme, light *(Land O Lakes* Cocoa
   Classics) 140
Coconut, shelled:
fresh, shredded or grated, 1 cup not packed 283
canned, flaked *(Angel Flake)*, 2 tbsp. 70
packaged, flaked *(Angel Flake)*, 2 tbsp. 70
packaged, shredded *(Baker's* Premium), 2 tbsp. 60
Coconut cream, canned *(Coco Casa)*, 3 tbsp. 170
Coconut milk, canned *(Taste of Thai)*, ¼ cup 110
Coconut nectar *(R.W. Knudsen)*, 8 fl. oz. 140
Cod, meat only, baked or broiled, 4 oz. 119
Cod, canned, Atlantic, w/liquid, 4 oz. 119
Cod, dried, Atlantic, salted, 1 oz. 81
Cod entree, frozen:
breaded *(Mrs. Paul's* Premium), 4.25-oz. piece 250
breaded *(Van de Kamp's* Light), 3.98-oz. piece 220

Coffee, brewed, 6 fl. oz. 4
Coffee, iced, canned *(Jamaican Gold),* 11 oz. 140
Coffee substitute:
(Natural Touch Kaffree Roma), 1 tsp. 10
(Natural Touch Roma Cappuccino), 3 tbsp. 50
(Postum Instant), 1 tsp. 10
Collard greens:
fresh, boiled, drained, chopped, ½ cup 17
canned *(Allens/Sunshine),* ½ cup 30
frozen, chopped, boiled, drained, ½ cup 31
Cookie:
all varieties *(Barbara's* Fat Free), 2 pieces, .9 oz. 80
almond *(Archway* Crescents), 2 pieces, .8 oz. 100
almond *(Frieda's),* 2 pieces, 1 oz. 170
almond *(Stella D'Oro* Breakfast Treats), .8-oz. piece 100
animal *(Barbara's Snackimals),* 8 pieces, 1.1 oz. 120
animal *(Sunshine),* 14 pieces, 1.1 oz. 140
anisette *(Stella D'Oro* Sponge), 2 pieces, 1 oz. 90
apple 'n raisin *(Archway* Gourmet), .9-oz. piece 110
apricot delight *(Health Valley* Nonfat), 3 pieces 100
arrowroot *(National),* 2-oz. piece 20
biscotti, all varieties *(Health Valley),* 2 pieces, 1.1 oz. . . . 120
biscottini cashews *(Stella D'Oro),* .7-oz. piece 110
blueberry *(Fruitastic* Bar), 1 bar 40
brown edge wafer *(Nabisco),* 5 pieces, 1 oz. 140
butter *(Peek Freans* Petit Beurre), 4 pieces, 1 oz. 130
butter *(Pepperidge Farm Chessman),* 3 pieces, .9 oz. . . . 120
butter *(Sunshine),* 5 pieces, 1.1 oz. 140
butter, frosted *(Land O Lakes),* 2 pieces, .9 oz. 120
butternut *(Archway* Gourmet), .9-oz. piece 120
carrot cake *(Archway* Gourmet), 1-oz. piece 120
cashew nougat *(Archway),* 3 pieces, 1.1 oz. 170
chocolate:
   (Barbara's Double Dutch Crisp), .6-oz. piece 80
   (Pepperidge Farm Goldfish), 1.1 oz. 140
   brownie nut *(Pepperidge Farm),* 3 pieces, 1.1 oz. . . . 160
   covered *(Ritz),* 3 pieces, 1.1 oz. 150
   fudge *(Dare),* .7-oz. piece 97
   snaps *(Nabisco),* 7 pieces, 1.2 oz. 140
   wafer *(Nabisco* Famous), 5 pieces, 1.1 oz. 140

Cookie *(cont.)*
chocolate chip/chunk:
  (Archway), 1-oz. piece 130
  (Archway Ice Box), .8-oz. piece 120
  (Archway Gourmet Supreme), .9-oz. piece 120
  (Barbara's Crisp), .6-oz. piece 80
  (Chip-A-Roos), 3 pieces, 1.3 oz. 190
  (Chips Ahoy! Chewy), 3 pieces, 1.3 oz. 170
  (Chips Ahoy! Chunky), .6-oz. piece 80
  (Chips Deluxe), .5-oz. piece 80
  (Chips Deluxe Chocolate Lovers), .6-oz. piece 90
  (Dare), .5-oz. piece 77
  (Grandma's Big), 1.4-oz. piece 190
  (Pepperidge Farm Chesapeake), .9-oz. piece 140
  (Pepperidge Farm Nantucket), .9-oz. piece 130
  (Tastykake), 1.4-oz. piece 180
  bar *(Tastykake)*, 1.5-oz. bar 200
  drop *(Archway)*, .9-oz. piece 100
  fudge *(Grandma's* Big), 1.4-oz. piece 170
  fudge bar *(Grandma's)*, 1.5-oz. bar 190
  macadamia *(Pepperidge Farm* Sausalito), .9-oz.
    piece 140
  macadamia, soft *(Pepperidge Farm)*, .9-oz. piece . . . 130
  mini *(Sunshine)*, 5 pieces, 1.1 oz. 160
  rainbow *(Chips Deluxe)*, .6-oz. piece 80
  snaps *(Nabisco)*, 7 pieces, 1.1 oz. 150
  soft *(Chips Deluxe)*, .5-oz. piece 70
  soft *(Pepperidge Farm* Chunk), .9-oz. piece 130
  toffee *(Archway* Gourmet), 1-oz. piece 130
  toffee *(Pepperidge Farm* Charleston), .9-oz. piece . . . 130
  walnut *(Pepperidge Farm* Beacon Hill), .9-oz. piece . 130
chocolate sandwich:
  (Hydrox), 3 pieces, 1.1 oz. 150
  (Oreo), 3 pieces, 1.2 oz. 160
  (Oreo Double Stuf), 2 pieces, 1 oz. 140
  (Pepperidge Farm Bordeaux), 4 pieces, 1 oz. 130
  (Pepperidge Farm Lido), .6-oz. piece 90
  (Pepperidge Farm Milano), 3 pieces, 1.2 oz. 180
  double *(Pepperidge Farm* Milano), 2 pieces, 1 oz. . . . 150
  fudge coated *(Oreo)*, .75-oz. piece 110

hazelnut *(Pepperidge Farm Milano)*, 2 pieces, .9 oz. . 130
milk *(Pepperidge Farm Bordeaux)*, 3 pieces, 1.1 oz. . 160
mint *(Pepperidge Farm Brussels)*, 3 pieces, 1.3 oz. . 190
mint or orange *(Pepperidge Farm Milano)*, 2 pieces . 140
white fudge coated *(Oreo)*, .75-oz. piece 110
cinnamon honey *(Archway* Hearts), 3 pieces, 1.1 oz. . . . 110
cocoa, Dutch *(Archway)*, .8-oz. piece 100
cranberry bar *(Newtons* Fat Free), 2 pieces, 1 oz. 100
Danish *(Nabisco* Import), 5 pieces, 1.2 oz. 170
date delight *(Health Valley* Nonfat), 3 pieces 100
devil's food *(Archway* Fat Free), .7-oz. piece 70
fig *(Fig Newtons)*, 2 pieces, 1.1 oz. 110
fig *(Sunshine* Bar), 2 pieces, 1 oz. 110
fortune *(Frieda's)*, 4 pieces, 1 oz. 120
fortune *(La Choy)*, 4 pieces, 1 oz. 110
fruit bar *(Archway* Fat Free), .8-oz. piece 80
fruit bar, all flavors *(Barbara's)*, .7-oz. piece 60
fruit cake *(Archway)*, 3 pieces, 1.1 oz. 140
fruit and honey *(Archway)*, .9-oz. piece 100
fruit-filled, all flavors *(Archway)*, .9-oz. piece 100
fudge:
   (Stella D'Oro Swiss), 2 pieces, .9 oz. 130
   bits *(Grandma's)*, 9 pieces 170
   fudge filled *(Keebler* Truffles), 3 pieces, 1.2 oz. 180
   mint patties *(Sunshine)*, 2 pieces, .8 oz. 130
   nutty *(Grandma's* Big), 1.4-oz. piece 190
   sandwich *(Grandma's)*, 1 pkg. 240
ginger *(Dare Breaktime)*, .3-oz. piece 34
ginger *(Pepperidge Farm* Gingerman), 4 pieces, 1 oz. . . . 120
ginger snaps:
   (Archway), 5 pieces, 1.1 oz. 150
   (Archway Reduced Fat), 5 pieces, 1.1 oz. 150
   (Sunshine), 7 pieces, 1 oz. 130
   iced *(Archway)*, 5 pieces, 1.3 oz. 170
gingerbread, iced *(Archway)*, 3 pieces, 1.1 oz. 140
gingerbread, iced *(Sunshine)*, 5 pieces, 1 oz. 130
graham:
   (Nabisco), 8 pieces, 1 oz. 120
   (Pepperidge Farm Goldfish), 1.1 oz. 150
   amaranth *(Health Valley* Fat Free), 11 pieces, 1 oz. . 100

Cookie, graham *(cont.)*
    chocolate *(Keebler)*, 8 pieces, 1.1 oz. 140
    chocolate *(Nabisco* Pure), 3 pieces, 1.1 oz. 160
    cinnamon *(Honey Maid)*, 10 pieces, 1.1 oz. 140
    fudge dipped *(Sunshine)*, 4 pieces, 1.2 oz. 170
    honey *(Honey Maid)*, 8 pieces, 1 oz. 120
    honey *(Sunshine)*, 2 pieces, 1 oz. 120
granola *(Archway* Fat Free), 2 pieces, 1.1 oz. 100
granola, soft *(Grandma's* Bar), 1.5-oz. bar 180
hazelnut *(Pepperidge Farm)*, 3 pieces, 1.1 oz. 160
hermits *(Archway* Cookie Jar), .9-oz. piece 90
(Heyday Bar), .75-oz. bar 110
kichel *(Stella D'Oro* Low Sodium), 21 pieces, 1 oz. 150
lemon *(Sunshine* Coolers), 5 pieces, 1.1 oz. 140
lemon creme *(Dare)*, .7-oz. piece 95
lemon drop *(Archway)*, .8-oz. piece 90
lemon nuggets *(Archway* Fat Free), 4 pieces, 1.1 oz. . . . 110
lemon nut crunch *(Pepperidge Farm)*, 3 pieces, 1.1 oz. . 170
lemon snaps *(Archway)*, 5 pieces, 1.1 oz. 150
lemon or orange, frosty *(Archway)*, .9-oz. piece 110
macaroon, coconut *(Archway)*, .8-oz. piece 100
marshmallow:
    chocolate *(Mallomars)*, 2 pieces, .9 oz. 120
    chocolate *(Pinwheels)*, 1.1-oz. piece 130
    fudge puffs *(Nabisco)*, .75-oz. piece 90
    fudge twirls *(Nabisco)*, 1.1-oz. piece 130
mint sandwich *(Mystic Mint)*, .6-oz. piece 90
molasses:
    (Archway/Archway Old Fashioned), .9-oz. piece 100
    (Grandma's Old Time Big), 1.4-oz. piece 160
    crisps *(Pepperidge Farm)*, 5 pieces, 1.1 oz. 150
    dark *(Archway)*, 1-oz. piece 120
    drop, soft *(Archway)*, .8-oz. piece 90
molasses or oatmeal, iced *(Archway)*, 1-oz. piece 120
mud pie *(Archway)*, .9-oz. piece 110
nougat, nutty *(Archway)*, 3 pieces, 1.1 oz. 170
oatmeal:
    (Archway), .9-oz. piece 100
    (Barbara's Old Fashioned Crisp), .6-oz. piece 70
    (Dare Breaktime), .3-oz. piece 35

(Nabisco Family Favorites), .6-oz. piece 80
(Ruth's/Ruth's Golden), 1-oz. piece 120
(Sunshine Country), 3 pieces, 1.2 oz. 170
apple or date filled *(Archway)*, .9-oz. piece 100
apple spice *(Grandma's* Big), 1.4-oz. piece 170
crunch *(Archway* Gourmet), .9-oz. piece 120
iced *(Sunshine)*, 2 pieces, .9 oz. 120
Irish *(Pepperidge Farm)*, 3 pieces, 1 oz. 130
pecan *(Archway* Gourmet), 1-oz. piece 140
oatmeal raisin:
  (Archway), .9-oz. piece 110
(Little Debbie), 2 pieces, 1.3 oz. 170
  (Pepperidge Farm Soft), .9-oz. piece 110
  (Tastykake Bar), 1.5-oz. bar 190
  or raspberry *(Archway* Fat Free), 1.1-oz. piece 110
peanut *(Archway* Jumble), 1-oz. piece 130
peanut butter:
  (Archway), .75-oz. piece 100
  (Archway Jumble), .8-oz. piece 110
  (Archway Ol' Fashion Gourmet), .8-oz. piece 120
  (Archway Ruth's), .9-oz. piece 110
  (Grandma's Big), 1.4-oz. piece 190
  bits *(Grandma's)*, 9 pieces 150
  chocolate chip *(Grandma's* Bar), 1.5-oz. bar 210
  chocolate chip *(Grandma's* Big), 1¼-oz. piece 190
  golden *(Archway* Ruth's Gourmet), 1-oz. piece 120
  patties *(Nutter Butter)*, 5 pieces, 1.1 oz. 160
  sandwich *(Grandma's)*, 5 pieces 210
  sandwich *(Nutter Butter)*, 2 pieces, 1 oz. 130
pecan *(Archway* Ice Box), .8-oz. piece 120
pecan malted nougat *(Archway)*, 3 pieces, 1.1 oz. 160
pound cake *(Archway* Aunt Bea's), .9-oz. piece 100
prune pastry *(Stella D'Oro* Sodium Free), .7-oz. piece . . 90
pumpkin spice *(Archway)*, 3 pieces, 1.1 oz. 120
raisin *(Dare Sun•Maid)*, .5-oz. piece 52
raspberry *(Fruitastic* Bar), 1 bar 40
raspberry *(Newtons* Fat Free), 2 pieces, 1 oz. 100
raspberry nuggets *(Archway* Fat Free), 4 pieces, 1.1 oz. . 120
rocky road *(Archway* Gourmet), 1-oz. piece 130
sesame *(Stella D'Oro* Regina), 3 pieces, 1-oz. piece 150

Cookie *(cont.)*
shortbread:
    (Barbara's Traditional Crisp), .6-oz. piece 80
    (Lorna Doone), 4 pieces, 1 oz. 140
    (Pepperidge Farm), 2 pieces, .9 oz. 140
    (Simply Sandies), .5-oz. piece 80
    butter *(Dare)*, .5-oz. piece 63
    fudge striped *(Sunshine)*, 3 pieces, 1.1 oz. 160
    pecan *(Pecan Sandies)*, .6-oz. piece 80
    pecan *(Pepperidge Farm)*, 2 pieces, .9 oz. 140
spice, pfeffernuss *(Archway)*, 2 pieces, 1 oz. 100
sprinkles *(Dare Breaktime)*, .3-oz. piece 36
sugar *(Archway)*, .8-oz. piece 100
sugar *(Archway Fat Free)*, .7-oz. piece 70
sugar *(Pepperidge Farm)*, 3 pieces, 1.1 oz. 140
sugar drop, soft *(Archway)*, .8-oz. piece 90
sugar wafer *(Biscos)*, 8 pieces, 1 oz. 140
sugar wafer *(Sunshine)*, 3 pieces, .9 oz. 130
vanilla bits *(Grandma's)*, 9 pieces 150
vanilla sandwich *(Cookie Break)*, 3 pieces, 1.1 oz. . . . 160
vanilla sandwich *(Vienna Fingers)*, 2 pieces, 1 oz. . . . 130
vanilla wafer *(Nilla)*, 8 pieces, 1.1 oz. 140
wafer, all flavors *(Grandma's Value)*, 4 pieces 160
walnut, black *(Archway Ice Box)*, .8-oz. piece 120
walnut, nutty *(Archway)*, .9-oz. piece 120
windmill *(Archway Old Fashioned)*, .7-oz. piece 90
Cookie crumbs, see "Pie crust"
Cooking sauce, see specific listings
Coriander:
fresh, ¼ cup 1
dried, ground *(McCormick)*, ¼ tsp. 2
dried, seeds *(McCormick)*, ¼ tsp. 3
Corn, fresh:
(Dole), 1 medium ear, 3.2 oz. 80
kernels, boiled, drained, ½ cup 89
Corn, canned, ½ cup, except as noted:
baby *(Haddon House)* 30
kernel *(Del Monte)* 90
kernel *(Del Monte Supersweet Vac Pack)* 70
kernel *(Green Giant/Green Giant 50% Less Sodium)* 80

kernel *(Green Giant Niblets),* ⅓ cup 70
kernel *(Green Giant Niblets* No Salt/Sugar), ⅓ cup 60
kernel *(S&W)* 90
kernel *(Stokely/Stokely* No Salt) 90
kernel, white *(Green Giant* Shoepeg), ⅓ cup 80
kernel, white or gold and white *(Del Monte)* 80
kernel, w/peppers *(Del Monte* Fiesta) 50
kernel, w/peppers *(Green Giant Mexicorn),* ⅓ cup 60
kernel, w/peppers *(Stokely),* ⅓ cup 80
cream style *(Del Monte/Del Monte* No Salt) 90
cream style *(Del Monte* Supersweet/Supersweet No
  Salt) 60
cream style *(Green Giant)* 100
cream style *(S&W)* 100
cream style *(Seneca)* 80
cream style, white *(Del Monte)* 100
Corn, frozen:
on cob *(Green Giant* Extra Sweet), 1 ear 120
on cob *(Green Giant* Nibblers), 1 ear 70
on cob *(Green Giant* Niblets), 1 ear 160
on cob *(Ore-Ida* Mini-Gold), 1 ear 80
on cob *(Seneca),* 1 ear 140
kernel *(Green Giant Niblets),* ⅔ cup 80
kernel *(Green Giant Niblets* Extra Sweet), ⅔ cup 70
kernel *(Seneca),* ⅔ cup 90
kernel *(Stilwell),* ⅔ cup 80
kernel, white *(Green Giant* Extra Sweet), ⅔ cup 50
kernel, white *(Green Giant* Shoepeg), ¾ cup 100
kernel, white *(Green Giant* Harvest Fresh), ½ cup 70
cream style *(Green Giant),* ½ cup 110
in butter sauce *(Green Giant Niblets),* ⅔ cup 130
in butter sauce, white *(Green Giant),* ¾ cup 120
Corn bread, see "Bread mix" and "Bread, frozen"
Corn chips, puffs, and similar snacks, 1 oz., except
  as noted:
(Barrel O'Fun Chips), 1.1 oz. 160
(Dipsey Doodles) 160
(Fritos King Size/Original/Wild 'N Mild/Scoops) 160
(Old Dutch Chips), 1.1 oz. 170
all varieties *(Sunchips)* 140

Corn chips, puffs, and similar snacks *(cont.)*
barbecue *(Fritos)* 150
barbecue *(Old Dutch)*, 1.1 oz. 165
cheese *(Cheese Doodles)* 150
cheese *(Chee•tos* Cheesy Checkers/Crunchy/Curls) 150
cheese, hot *(Chee•tos* Flamin') 160
cheese, nacho *(Doodle Twisters)* 160
cheese balls *(Barrel O'Fun)*, 1.1 oz. 160
cheese balls *(Chee•tos)* 160
cheese balls or curls *(Planters* Cheez) 150
cheese curls *(Old Dutch* Crunchy) 130
cheese puffs *(Barbara's* Bakes) 160
cheese puffs *(Barrel O'Fun* Light), 1.1 oz. 125
cheese puffs *(Chee•tos)* 160
cheese puffs, all varieties *(Barbara's* 40% Less Fat) 140
cheese puffs, original or jalapeño *(Barbara's)* 150
cheese, cheddar, or ranch puffs *(No Fries)* 110
chili-cheese *(Fritos)* 160
multigrain *(Barbara's* Pinta Chips) 130
nacho cheese *(Chee•tos)* 160
tortilla:
　(Nachips) 150
　(No Fries Natural) 100
　(Old Dutch Restaurant) 140
　(Santitas Chips/Strips) 140
　(Tostitos Baked/Unsalted/Bite Size) 110
　(Tostitos Crispy Round) 150
　(Tostitos Restaurant) 130
　(Tostitos Restaurant Unsalted/Santa Fe Gold/Bite
　　Size) 140
　all varieties *(Doritos* Reduced Fat) 130
　all varieties *(Kettle Tias)* 140
　all varieties *(No Fries)*, 1.1 oz. 110
　all varieties, except spicy nacho and *Taco Bell* taco
　　supreme *(Doritos)* 140
　blue corn *(Barbara's)*, 1.1 oz. 140
　lime and chili *(Tostitos)* 150
　ranch *(Tostitos* Baked) 120
　salsa & cream cheese *(Tostitos)* 120
　spicy nacho *(Doritos)* 150

Taco Bell taco supreme *(Doritos)* 150
   tostados *(Old Dutch)*, 1.1 oz. 150
Corn flour, masa, 1 cup 416
Cornflake crumbs *(Kellogg's)*, 2 tbsp. 40
Corn grits, dry, ¼ cup:
(Goya) 180
(Jim Dandy) 170
(Jim Dandy Quick Grits) 160
iron-fortified *(Jim Dandy)* 140
white *(Quaker* Hominy) 140
white *(Quaker* Quick Hominy) 130
yellow *(Martha White)* 150
yellow *(Quaker* Quick Hominy) 120
Corn relish *(Nance's)*, 2 tbsp. 25
Corn soufflé, frozen *(Stouffer's)*, 4.8 oz. 170
Cornish hen:
roasted, half, dark meat *(Perdue)*, 6.6 oz. 300
roasted, half, white meat *(Perdue)*, 6.6 oz. 190
Cornmeal (see also "Corn flour" and "Polenta"):
(Frieda's), ¼ cup, 1.1 oz. 110
blue or hi-lysine *(Arrowhead Mills)*, ¼ cup 130
blue and red *(Frieda's)*, ½ cup 214
masa harina *(Quaker* Enriched), ¼ cup 110
masa harina *(Quaker* Preparada Para Tortillas), ⅓ cup . 160
self-rising, 3 tbsp.:
   degerminated *(Jim Dandy)* 110
   stone-ground *(Cabin Home/Pine Mountain)* 110
   white, regular or degerminated *(Aunt Jemima)* 90
white or yellow *(Albers)*, 3 tbsp. 110
white or yellow *(Arrowhead Mills)*, ¼ cup 120
Cornstarch *(Argo/Kingsford)*, 1 tbsp. 30
Couscous, cooked, ½ cup 101
Couscous mix:
almond chicken, vegetarian *(Casbah)*, 1 cont. 160
asparagus au gratin *(Casbah)*, 1 cont. 150
cheddar, broccoli, creamy *(Casbah)*, 1 cont. 130
pilaf *(Casbah)*, 1 oz. 100
tomato Parmesan *(Casbah)*, 1 cont. 170
Cowpeas (see also "Black-eyed peas"):
fresh, boiled, drained, ½ cup 79

Cowpeas *(cont.)*

frozen, boiled, drained, ½ cup 112
mature, boiled, ½ cup 100

Crab, meat only, 4 oz.:

Alaska king, boiled, poached, or steamed 110
blue, boiled, poached, or steamed 116
Dungeness, boiled, poached, or steamed 125
queen, boiled, poached, or steamed 130

Crab, canned, Dungeness *(S&W)*, ⅓ cup, 3 oz. 80

"Crab," imitation, frozen or refrigerated:

(Peter Pan), 3 oz. 70
flaked *(Seafest)*, 3 oz., ½ cup 100
flaked, chunk or "leg" *(Louis Kemp Crab Delights)*,
   3 oz. 80

Crabapple, canned:

(S&W), 1 piece 35
spiced *(Apple Time)*, 1 piece, 1.1 oz. 40

Cracker:

(Barbara's Rite Lite), 5 pieces, .5 oz. 55
butter/butter flavor:
   (Hi-Ho), 9 pieces, 1.1 oz. 160
   (Ritz/Ritz Low Sodium), 5 pieces, .6 oz. 80
   (Ritz Air Crisps), 24 pieces, 1 oz. 140
   (Ritz Bits), 48 pieces, 1.1 oz. 160
   (Town House), 5 pieces, .6 oz. 80
   thins *(Pepperidge Farm)*, 4 pieces, .5 oz. 70
cheese:
   (Appeteasers Original), 1 oz. 130
   (Nips), 29 pieces, 1.1 oz. 150
   (Nips Air Crisps), 32 pieces, 1 oz. 130
   (Tid-Bit), 32 pieces, 1.1 oz. 150
   Parmesan *(Goldfish)*, 60 pieces, 1.1 oz. 140
cheese, cheddar:
   (Better Cheddars), 22 pieces, 1.1 oz. 150
   (Better Cheddars Reduced Fat), 24 pieces, 1.1 oz. . . . 140
   (Cheez-It), 27 pieces, 1.1 oz. 160
   (Cheez-It Reduced Fat), 30 pieces, 1.1 oz. 130
   (Frito-Lay), 1 pkg. 220
   (Goldfish), 55 pieces, 1.1 oz. 140
   bacon *(Chee•tos)*, 1 pkg. 200

cheese sandwich *(Little Debbie)*, 1.4 oz. 200
cheese sandwich *(Ritz)*, 1.4-oz. pkg. 210
croissant *(Carr's)*, 3 pieces, .5 oz. 70
flatbread *(Lavosh Hawaii* Classic), 8 pieces, 1 oz. 120
flatbread, all varieties *(J.J. Flats)*, .5-oz. piece 50
(Goldfish Original), 55 pieces, 1.1 oz. 140
matzo *(Manischewitz* Unsalted/Everything!/Rye), 1 oz. . . 110
melba rounds, all varieties *(Old London)*, 5 pieces,
   .5 oz. 60
melba toast, all varieties *(Devonsheer)*, 3 pieces, .5 oz. . . 50
multigrain *(Hi-Ho)*, 9 pieces, 1.1 oz. 160
multigrain *(Wheat Thins)*, 17 pieces, 1.1 oz. 130
(Munch 'ems), 30 pieces, 1.1 oz. 130
oat *(Harvest Crisps)*, 13 pieces, 1.1 oz. 140
onion, French *(Wheatables)*, 29 pieces, 1.1 oz. 130
peanut butter *(Handi-Snacks)*, 1.1-oz. piece 180
peanut butter sandwich, cheese *(Little Debbie)*, 1 pkg. . 200
peanut butter sandwich, cheese or toast *(Planters)*,
   1 pkg. 190
peanut butter sandwich, toast *(Little Debbie)*, 1 pkg. . . . 190
pizza, all varieties *(Health Valley)*, 6 pieces 50
ranch *(Munch 'ems)*, 33 pieces, 1.1 oz. 130
rice, bran *(Health Valley)*, 6 pieces, 1 oz. 110
salsa *(Munch 'ems)*, 28 pieces, 1.1 oz. 130
saltines *(Krispy)*, 5 pieces, .5 oz. 60
saltines *(Zesta)*, 5 pieces, .5 oz. 60
sesame *(Breton)*, 10 pieces, 1.5 oz. 220
sesame cheese *(Twigs)*, 15 pieces, 1.1 oz. 150
(Sociables), 7 pieces, .5 oz. 80
soup and oyster *(Oysterettes)*, .5 oz. 60
vegetable *(Vegetable Thins)*, 14 pieces, 1.1 oz. 160
vegetable *(Vivant)*, 3 pieces, .5 oz. 70
water or soda:
   (Breton), 10 pieces, 1.5 oz. 210
   (Breton Light), 10 pieces, 1.5 oz. 200
   (Cabaret), 10 pieces, 1.7 oz. 230
   (Carr's Table Water), 5 pieces, .6 oz. 70
   (Vivant), 10 pieces, 1.5 oz. 210
   cracked pepper *(Carr's Table Water)*, 5 pieces,
      .6 oz. 70

Cracker, water or soda *(cont.)*
sesame *(Breton)*, 10 pieces, .5 oz. 220
wheat:
  (Stoned Wheat Thins), 2 pieces 60
  (Triscuit), 7 pieces, 1.1 oz. 140
  (Waverly), 5 pieces, .5 oz. 70
  (Wheat Thins Air Crisps), 24 pieces 130
  (Wheatables), 26 pieces, 1.1 oz. 150
  (Wheatsworth), 5 pieces, .6 oz. 80
  all varieties *(Barbara's* Wheatines), .5-oz. large
    square 60
  herb, garden *(Triscuit)*, 6 pieces, 1 oz. 130
  and rye *(Triscuit* Deli), 7 pieces, 1.1 oz. 140
  whole *(Hi-Ho)*, 9 pieces, 1.1 oz. 150
  whole *(Krispy)*, 5 pieces, .5 oz. 60
  whole, all varieties *(Health Valley)*, 5 pieces . . . 50
Cranberry, fresh, raw, whole, ½ cup 23
Cranberry, dried *(Frieda's)*, ⅓ cup, 1.4 oz. . . . 120
Cranberry beans:
boiled, ½ cup 120
canned, w/liquid, ½ cup 108
Cranberry drink, 8 fl. oz.:
(Tropicana Punch) 140
(Tropicana Ruby Red) 120
juice cocktail *(Seneca)* 140
Cranberry drink blends, 8 fl. oz.:
hibiscus *(R.W. Knudsen)* 120
raspberry *(R.W. Knudsen)* 140
raspberry-strawberry *(Tropicana Twister)* 120
Cranberry juice, 8 fl. oz., except as noted:
(After the Fall Cape Cod) 100
(After the Fall Nantucket) 60
(Apple & Eve Naturally Cranberry) 120
(Ocean Spray Cocktail), 6 fl. oz. 100
(Snapple Royale), 10 fl. oz. 150
Cranberry juice blends, 8 fl. oz., except as noted:
apple *(Cranapple)* 160
apple *(Dole)* 120
apple *(Snapple)*, 12 fl. oz. 200
apricot *(Cranicot)* 160

grape *(Apple & Eve)*, 10 fl. oz. 175
kiwi or mango *(After the Fall)* 100
punch *(Crantastic)* 150
raspberry *(After the Fall)* 90
strawberry *(Ocean Spray)* 140
Cranberry nectar *(Santa Cruz)*, 8 fl. oz. 110
Cranberry sauce, whole or jellied *(S&W)*, ¼ cup 100
Crayfish, mixed species, meat only:
wild, boiled or steamed, 4 oz. 100
farmed, boiled or steamed, 4 oz. 99
Cream, dairy pack (see also "Cream, sour"):
half-and-half *(America's Choice)*, 2 tbsp. 40
light, coffee or table, 1 tbsp. 29
whipping, light, 1 tbsp. or 2 tbsp. whipped 44
whipping, heavy, 1 tbsp. or 2 tbsp. whipped 52
Cream, sour, 2 tbsp.:
(Heluva Good) 60
(Sealtest) 60
light *(Heluva* Good) 40
light *(Land O Lakes)* 35
nondairy, plain or flavored *(Sour Supreme)* 50
nonfat *(Breakstone's/Sealtest Free)* 35
nonfat *(Heluva* Good) 20
Cream topping, 2 tbsp.:
(Cool Whip Extra Creamy) 30
(Cool Whip Lite) 20
(Cool Whip Non-dairy) 25
(Kraft Real/Whipped Topping) 20
(Pet Whip) 30
mix* *(Dream Whip)* 20
Creamer, nondairy, 1 tbsp., except as noted:
(Coffee-mate) 20
(Coffee-mate Fat Free/Lite) 10
(Rich's Coffee Rich) 25
(Rich's Farm Rich) 20
(Rich's Farm Rich Fat Free/Light) 10
powder *(Cremora/Cremora* Fat Free/Lite), 1 tsp. 10
Cress, water, see "Watercress"
Croissant, 1 piece:
butter *(Awrey's)*, 1.5 oz. 140

Croissant *(cont.)*
butter *(Awrey's)*, 2 oz. 190
butter *(Awrey's Tip-to-Tip)* 290
dill and onion *(Awrey's)* 210
margarine *(Awrey's Tip-to-Tip)* 140
margarine, sandwich *(Awrey's)*, 1.8 oz. 180
margarine, sandwich *(Awrey's)*, 2.5 oz. 250
frozen *(Sara Lee* Original) 170
Crookneck squash, ½ cup:
fresh, sliced, boiled, drained 18
canned, cut, yellow *(Allens/Sunshine)* 16
Croutons (see also "Salad toppers"):
all varieties *(Arnold* Crispy), 2 tbsp. 30
all varieties *(Brownberry)*, 2 tbsp. 30
all varieties *(Old London* Restaurant Style), 2 tbsp. 30
Cucumber, w/peel:
1 medium, 8¼ long 38
sliced, ½ cup 7
hothouse or Japanese *(Frieda's)*, ⅔ cup, 3 oz. 10
Cucuzza squash *(Frieda's)*, ¾ cup, 3 oz. 10
Cumin seeds, ground, 1 tsp. 8
Currant, dried, Zante *(S&W)*, ¼ cup 130
Curry powder, 1 tbsp. 20
Curry sauce, cooking:
(Kylin Thai), ¼ cup 25
Masala *(Shahi* Cream/Curry), ¼ cup 50
Cusk, meat only, baked or broiled, 4 oz. 127
Cuttlefish, meat only, boiled or steamed, 4 oz. 179

FOOD AND MEASURE	CALORIES

Daikon, see "Radish, Oriental"
Dairy Queen/Brazier, 1 serving:
DQ Homestyle burgers:
    cheeseburger 340
    cheeseburger, deluxe double 540
    cheeseburger, double 540
    cheeseburger w/bacon, double 610
    hamburger 290
    Ultimate burger 670
sandwiches:
    chicken breast fillet, breaded 430
    chicken fillet, grilled 310
    hot dog, plain 240
    hot dog, w/chili and cheese 330
chicken strip basket, w/gravy, toast, and fries 1,000
side dishes:
    fries, large 440
    fries, medium 350
    onion rings 320
desserts and shakes:
    banana split 510
    Blizzard:
        chocolate chip cookie dough, medium 950
        chocolate chip cookie dough, small 660
        chocolate sandwich cookie, medium 640
        chocolate sandwich cookie, small 520
    Buster Bar 450
    cone, chocolate, medium 340
    cone, chocolate, small 240
    cone, chocolate-dipped, medium 490
    cone, chocolate-dipped, small 340
    cone, vanilla, large 410
    cone, vanilla, medium 330

Dairy Queen/Brazier, desserts and shakes *(cont.)*

cone, vanilla, small 230
DQ cake, undecorated, 8˝ round, 1/8 cake 340
DQ fudge bar 50
DQ Lemon Freez'r, 1/2 cup 80
DQ sandwich 150
DQ Treatzza Pizza, 1/8 pie:
    Heath or strawberry-banana 180
    M&M's 190
DQ vanilla orange bar 60
Dilly bar, chocolate 210
Fudge Cake Supreme 890
malt, chocolate, medium 880
malt, chocolate, small 650
Misty slush, medium 290
Misty slush, small 220
Peanut Buster parfait 730
shake, chocolate, medium 770
shake, chocolate, small 560
soft-serve, *DQ,* chocolate, 1/2 cup 150
soft-serve, *DQ,* vanilla, 1/2 cup 140
Starkiss 80
strawberry shortcake 430
sundae, chocolate, medium 400
sundae, chocolate, small 280
yogurt, *Breeze:*
    Heath, medium 710
    Heath, small 470
    strawberry, medium 460
    strawberry, small 320
yogurt, frozen:
    DQ nonfat, 1/2 cup 100
    medium cup 230
    cone 260
    strawberry sundae 280
Dandelion greens, raw *(Frieda's),* 2 cups, 3 oz. 40
Danish, 1 piece:
all varieties *(Awrey's* Petite) 130
apple or cinnamon swirl *(Awrey's)* 300
cheese *(Awrey's)* 300

cheese *(Tastykake* Pocket) 410
cheese, cherry or lemon *(Awrey's* Marquise) 350
strawberry *(Awrey's)* 300
Date, dried, pitted:
(Dole), ½ cup 280
(Sonoma), 5–6 pieces, 1.4 oz. 110
chopped *(Dole),* ½ cup 230
Date nut pastry *(Awrey's),* 1 piece 130
Delicata squash *(Frieda's),* ¾ cup, 3 oz. 30
Dessert mix, chilled, no-bake:
banana cream *(Betty Crocker),* ⅑ dessert* 250
chocolate French silk *(Betty Crocker),* ⅛ dessert* 270
coconut cream *(Betty Crocker),* ⅑ dessert* 290
cookies 'n creme *(Betty Crocker),* ⅙ dessert* 360
Sunkist lemon supreme *(Betty Crocker),* ⅑ dessert* . . . 320
Dill dip *(Marie's),* 2 tbsp. 190
Dill seed, 1 tsp. 6
Dill weed:
fresh, ½ cup loosely packed 2
dried, 1 tsp. 3
Dock, boiled, drained, 4 oz. 23
Dolphinfish, meat only, baked or broiled, 4 oz. 124
Donut, 1 piece, except as noted:
(Tastykake Assorted) 180
plain *(Awrey's),* 1.5-oz. piece 170
plain *(Awrey's),* 2-oz. piece 240
plain *(Hostess)* 140
blueberry *(Hostess)* 210
chocolate frosted/iced:
   (Awrey's), 1.75-oz. piece 200
   (Awrey's), 2.5-oz. piece 300
   (Hostess) 180
   chocolate *(Awrey's),* 1.75-oz. piece 190
   chocolate *(Awrey's),* 2.5-oz. piece 280
   custard Bismark *(Awrey's)* 350
   rich *(Tastykake)* 270
   rich, mini *(Tastykake),* 4 pieces 270
   ring *(Awrey's)* 350
   sour creme *(Awrey's)* 430
cinnamon *(Tastykake* Assorted) 210

Donut *(cont.)*
coconut top *(Awrey's)* 210
crunch *(Awrey's)* 280
crunch top *(Awrey's)* 160
glazed *(Hostess)* 270
glazed, honey, devil's food or ring *(Awrey's)* 310
glazed, orange *(Tastykake)* 220
glazed, sour creme *(Awrey's)* 420
honey wheat *(Tastykake)* 230
honey wheat, mini *(Tastykake)*, 6 pieces 280
powdered sugar:
   (Awrey's), 1.5-oz. piece 170
   (Awrey's), 2.25-oz. piece 390
   (Tastykake Assorted) 210
   cinnamon *(Hostess)* 150
   jelly Bismark *(Awrey's)* 320
   mini *(Tastykake)*, 6 pieces 290
raspberry filled *(Hostess O's)* 230
sour creme, plain *(Awrey's)* 370
sprinkle topped *(Awrey's)* 160
vanilla iced *(Awrey's Long John)* 380
vanilla iced, jelly Bismark *(Awrey's)* 320
white, iced *(Awrey's)* 200
Dressing, see "Salad dressing" and specific listings
Drum, freshwater, meat only, baked or broiled, 4 oz. . . . 173
Duck, domesticated, roasted:
meat w/skin, 4 oz. 382
meat only, 4 oz. 228
Dumpling squash, sweet *(Frieda's)*, ¾ cup, 3 oz. 30

E

FOOD AND MEASURE   **CALORIES**

Eclair, chocolate, frozen *(Rich's),* 1 piece 190
Eel, meat only:
raw, 4 oz. 209
baked, broiled, or microwaved, 4 oz. 268
Egg, chicken:
raw, whole, 1 large 75
raw, white only, 1 large 17
cooked, hard-boiled, chopped, 1 cup 210
Egg, quail, 1 egg 14
Egg, substitute or imitation, ¼ cup:
(Egg Beaters) 30
(Morningstar Farms Better'n Eggs) 20
(Morningstar Farms Scramblers) 35
(Second Nature) 40
Egg breakfast, frozen, 1 pkg.:
burrito, see "Burrito, breakfast"
omelet, ham and cheese *(Weight Watchers)* 220
scrambled:
   (Great Starts Low Fat) 240
   and bacon *(Great Starts)* 290
   and Canadian bacon *(Great Starts* Low Cholesterol/
     Fat) 240
   w/home fries *(Great Starts)* 200
   and pancakes *(Great Starts* Low Cholesterol/Fat) . . . 220
   and sausage *(Great Starts)* 360
Egg roll, frozen:
chicken *(Chun King/La Choy* Mini), 6 rolls 210
chicken *(Chun King* Restaurant Style), 3-oz. roll 190
chicken *(La Choy* Restaurant Style), 3-oz. roll 170
chicken, sweet and sour, or pork *(La Choy* Restaurant
   Style), 3-oz. roll 220
pork and shrimp *(Chun King/La Choy* Mini), 6 rolls 210
pork and shrimp *(La Choy* Bite Size), 12 rolls 210

Egg roll *(cont.)*
shrimp *(Chun King/La Choy* Mini), 6 rolls 190
shrimp *(Chun King/La Choy* Restaurant Style), 3-oz.
  roll 180
vegetable w/lobster *(La Choy* Mini), 6 rolls 190
" **'Egg' roll, vegetarian,** frozen *(Worthington),* 1 roll . . . 180
Egg roll wrapper *(Frieda's),* 2 pieces, 1.7 oz. 130
Eggnog, dairy, ½ cup:
(Crowley) 190
(Crowley Light) 120
(Crowley Nonfat) 130
Eggplant, fresh:
raw, trimmed, 1 pieces, ½ cup 11
boiled, drained, 1 cubes, ½ cup 13
Eggplant, Japanese, fresh *(Frieda's),* ⅔ cup, 3 oz. 20
Eggplant appetizer, in jars:
(Progresso Caponata), 2 tbsp. 25
roasted *(Peloponnese),* 2 tbsp. 25
Eggplant entree, frozen:
cutlets *(Celentano),* 5 oz. 210
parmigiana *(Celentano* 14 oz.), ½ pkg. 320
parmigiana *(Mrs. Paul's),* ½ cup 220
rollettes *(Celentano* Great Choice), 10 oz. 330
Eggplant pickle relish *(Patak's* Brinjal), 1 tbsp. 60
Elderberry, fresh, ½ cup 53
Empanadilla, frozen:
plain *(Goya),* 2 pieces 380
pizza flavor *(Goya),* 2 pieces 370
Enchilada, canned *(Gebhardt),* 2 pieces 260
Enchilada dinner, frozen:
beef *(Banquet* Extra Helping), 15.65 oz. 610
beef *(Swanson),* 1 pkg. 500
beef or cheese *(Patio),* 12 oz. 370
beef, 4 *(Patio* Chili 'N Beans), 15.5 oz. 540
beef, 2, and 2 cheese *(Patio* Chili 'N Beans), 15.5 oz. . . 610
chicken *(Patio),* 12 oz. 400
chicken, supreme *(Healthy Choice),* 11.3 oz. 300
Enchilada entree, frozen:
beef *(Banquet),* 11 oz. 370
beef, and tamale *(Banquet),* 11 oz. 400

beef or cheese *(Patio Family)*, 2 pieces, w/sauce 210
cheese or combo *(Banquet)*, 11 oz. 360
chicken *(Banquet)*, 11 oz. 350
chicken Suiza *(Healthy Choice)*, 10 oz. 280
Enchilada sauce, ¼ cup:
(Chi-Chi's) 30
(Gebhardt) 35
(La Victoria) 20
(Rosarita) 25
all varieties *(Old El Paso)* 30
green *(Las Palmas)* 25
Enchilada seasoning mix:
(Durkee), 1½ tsp. 10
(Lawry's), 2 tsp. 20
(Old El Paso), 2 tsp. 10
Endive, chopped, ½ cup 4
Endive, Belgian, see "Chicory, witloof"
Entree mix, frozen *(Green Giant Create A Meal!)*:
Alfredo, creamy, 2 cups[1] 210
Alfredo, creamy, 1¼ cups[2] 380
broccoli stir-fry, 2⅓ cups[1] 120
broccoli stir-fry, 1⅓ cups[2] 290
cheddar, creamy, 1¾ cups[1] 200
cheddar, creamy, 1½ cups[2] 290
cheese and herb primavera, 1¾ cups[1] 200
cheese and herb primavera, 1¼ cups[2] 330
chicken noodle, creamy, 1½ cups[1] 200
chicken noodle, creamy, 1¼ cups[2] 350
garlic herb, 2⅓ cups[1] 220
garlic herb, 1¼ cups[2] 340
lemon herb, 1½ cups[1] 210
lemon herb, 1½ cups[2] 380
lo mein, 2⅓ cups[1] 170
lo mein, 1¼ cups[2] 320
mushroom and wine, 1¾ cups[1] 210
mushroom and wine, 1¼ cups[2] 390

[1] As packaged.
[2] Prepared according to package directions, with meat and oil.

Entree mix, frozen *(cont.)*

sweet and sour, 1¾ cups[1]	130
sweet and sour, 1¼ cups[2]	290
Szechuan, 1¾ cups[1]	170
Szechuan, 1¼ cups[2]	340
teriyaki, 1¾ cups[1]	90
teriyaki, 1¼ cups[2]	240
vegetable almond stir-fry, 1¾ cups[1]	160
vegetable almond stir-fry, 1⅓ cups[2]	320
vegetable stew, hearty, 1¼ cups[1]	130
vegetable stew, hearty, 1¼ cups[2]	280
Eppaw, ½ cup	75

Escarole, see "Endive"

[1] *As packaged.*
[2] *Prepared according to package directions, with meat and oil.*

F

Fajita entree, frozen, chicken *(Healthy Choice* Fiesta),
    7 oz. 260
Fajita mix:
(Old El Paso), 2 pieces* 330
chicken *(Cafe Perdue* Meal Kit), 2 pieces* 300
Fajita sauce:
(S&W Southwestern), 1 tbsp. 10
skillet *(Lawry's)*, 2 tbsp. 15
Fajita seasoning mix:
(Lawry's), 2 tsp. 15
(Old El Paso), 1 tbsp. 30
beef *(Durkee* Easy), ⅙ pkg. 15
Falafel mix *(Fantastic Falafil)*, ½ cup 250
Farina, whole-grain (see also "Cereal"), cooked, 1 cup . 116
Fat, see specific listings
Fava beans, see "Broad beans"
Feijoa, raw *(Frieda's)*, 5 oz. 70
Fennel, bulb *(Frieda's)*, ¾ cup, 3 oz. 25
Fennel seeds, 1 tsp. 7
Fenugreek seeds, 1 tsp. 12
Fettuccine, refrigerated:
(Contadina), 1¼ cups 240
artichoke *(Tutta Pasta)*, 2 oz. 190
spinach *(Contadina)*, 1¼ cups 260
squid, black *(Tutta Pasta)*, 2 oz. 180
Fettuccine entree, frozen:
Alfredo *(Banquet)*, 9.5 oz. 350
Alfredo *(Healthy Choice)*, 8 oz. 250
Alfredo *(Marie Callender* Supreme), 1 cup, 6.5 oz. 450
Alfredo, w/broccoli *(Weight Watchers)*, 8.5 oz. 230
Alfredo, and garlic bread *(Marie Callender)*, 14 oz. . . . 800
w/broccoli, chicken *(Marie Callender)*, 1 cup, 6.5 oz. . . 410
chicken, see "Chicken entree"

Fettuccine entree, frozen *(cont.)*
primavera *(Marie Callender)*, 1 cup, 7 oz. 430
primavera *(Stouffer's)*, 10 oz. 430
Fettuccine entree mix, w/basil sauce *(Knorr* Cup),
  1 pkg. 220
Fig:
fresh, 1 large, 2.3 oz. 47
fresh, Calimyrna *(Frieda's)*, 1 oz. 23
canned, Kadota, in heavy syrup *(Oregon)*, ½ cup 130
Fig, dried:
California, 4 figs, 2 oz. 143
Calimyrna or mission *(Blue Ribbon/SunMaid)*, ¼ cup . . . 110
Filbert:
dried, 1 oz. 179
dry-roasted, salted or unsalted, 1 oz. 188
Finnan haddie, see "Haddock"
Fish, see specific listings
"Fish," vegetarian:
frozen *(Worthington)*, 2 fillets 180
mix *(Loma Linda* Ocean Platter), ⅓ cup 90
Fish batter mix, see "Fish seasoning and coating mix"
Fish dinner, frozen (see also specific fish listings):
battered portions, w/chips *(Swanson)*, 1 pkg. 490
fisherman's platter *(Swanson Hungry-Man)*, 1 pkg. 650
herb-baked *(Healthy Choice)*, 10.9 oz. 360
lemon pepper *(Healthy Choice)*, 10.7 oz. 320
Fish entree, frozen (see also specific fish listings):
(Van de Kamp's Fish 'n Fries), 6.5 oz. 380
baked, w/shells *(Lean Cuisine)*, 9 oz. 260
cakes *(Mrs. Paul's)*, 2 pieces 200
and chips *(Swanson* Lunch and More), 1 pkg. 350
fillets, baked:
  (Van de Kamp's Crisp & Healthy), 2 pieces 150
  garlic and pepper *(Mrs. Paul's/Van de Kamp's)*,
    1 piece 150
  lemon pepper *(Mrs. Paul's/Van de Kamp's)*, 1 piece . 140
fillets, battered:
  (Gorton's), 2 pieces 280
  (Mrs. Paul's), 1 piece 170
  (Van de Kamp's), 1 piece 180

lemon pepper *(Gorton's)*, 2 pieces 250
fillets, breaded, 2 pieces, except as noted:
   (Gorton's Crunchy) 270
   (Mrs. Paul's) 240
   (Mrs. Paul's Crisp & Healthy) 150
   (Van de Kamp's) 280
   cornmeal *(Mrs. Paul's/Van de Kamp's)*, 1 piece . . . 180
   garlic and herb *(Gorton's* Crunchy) 250
   hot and spicy *(Gorton's* Crunchy) 250
   potato *(Gorton's)* 290
   Southern fried *(Gorton's* Crunchy) 270
fillets, grilled, 1 piece:
   all varieties *(Mrs. Paul's/Van de Kamp's)* 130
   Italian herb *(Gorton's)* 130
   lemon pepper *(Gorton's)* 120
grilled, w/vegetables *(Lean Cuisine* Cafe Classics),
   $8^{7}/_{8}$ oz. 170
portions:
   battered *(Gorton's)*, 1 piece 160
   battered *(Van de Kamp's)*, 2 pieces 350
   breaded *(Mrs. Paul's)*, 2 pieces 190
   breaded *(Van de Kamp's)*, 3 pieces 330
sticks *(Banquet)*, 6.6 oz. 290
sticks, battered *(Gorton's)*, 5 pieces 290
sticks, battered *(Mrs. Paul's)*, 6 pieces 240
sticks, battered *(Van de Kamp's)*, 6 pieces 260
sticks, breaded, 6 pieces:
   (Gorton's Crunchy) 250
   (Gorton's Value Pack) 220
   (Mrs. Paul's) 200
   (Mrs. Paul's Value Pack) 210
   (Mrs. Paul's/Van de Kamp's Crisp & Healthy) 180
   (Van de Kamp's) 290
   (Van de Kamp's Snack/Value Pack) 260
   potato *(Gorton's)* 220
Fish seasoning, seafood *(Old Bay)*, ½tsp. 0
Fish seasoning and coating mix:
(Shake'n Bake), ¼ pkt. 70
lemon butter *(Durkee/French's* Roasting Bag), ¼ pkg. . . 30
Flatfish, see "Flounder" and "Sole"

Flavor enhancer, all varieties *(Ac'cent),* ¼ tsp. 0
Flax seeds *(Arrowhead Mills),* 3 tbsp. 140
Flounder, meat only:
fresh, baked or broiled, 4 oz. 133
frozen *(Van de Kamp's),* 4 oz. 110
Flounder entree, fillets, frozen:
breaded *(Mrs. Paul's* Premium), 2.9-oz. piece 170
breaded *(Van de Kamp's* Light), 3.98-oz. piece 230
Flour, see "Wheat flour" and other specific listings
Frankfurter, 1 link, except as noted:
(Boar's Head) 150
(Hormel 10), 1.6 oz. 140
(Hormel 8/Big 8), 2 oz. 180
(Hormel Light & Lean 97), 1.6 oz. 45
(Oscar Mayer Wieners) 150
(Oscar Mayer Wieners Light) 110
(Oscar Mayer Big & Juicy Wieners) 240
beef *(Boar's Head* Giant) 160
beef *(Boar's Head* Lite) 90
beef *(Hebrew National* 8 oz.) 140
beef *(Hebrew National* Quarter Pound/Jumbo) 350
beef *(Oscar Mayer)* 140
beef *(Oscar Mayer* Light) 110
beef *(Oscar Mayer Big & Juicy* Deli), 2.7 oz. 230
beef *(Wranglers)* 170
cocktail *(Hormel),* 5 links 160
cocktail beef *(Hebrew National),* 4 links 180
cheese *(Wranglers)* 170
hot and spicy *(Oscar Mayer Big & Juicy)* 220
smoked *(Wranglers)* 170
turkey, see "Turkey frankfurter"
"Frankfurter," vegetarian, 1 link:
(NewMenu VegiDog) 45
canned *(Loma Linda* Big Franks) 110
canned *(Loma Linda* Big Franks Low Fat) 80
canned *(Loma Linda* Linketts) 70
canned *(Worthington* Super-Links) 110
frozen *(Loma Linda* Corn) 200
frozen *(Morningstar Farms* Deli Franks) 110
frozen *(Natural Touch* Vege) 100

refrigerated, chili *(Yves Veggie Cuisine Dogs)* 70
French toast, frozen, 2 pieces:
(Downyflake) 260
cinnamon swirl *(Downyflake)* 270
regular or cinnamon swirl *(Aunt Jemima)* 240
French toast breakfast, frozen, 1 pkg.:
cinnamon swirl *(Great Starts)* 440
w/sausage *(Great Starts)* 410
sticks, w/syrup *(Great Starts)* 320
Frosting, ready-to-spread, 2 tbsp.:
all flavors *(Betty Crocker Creamy Deluxe)* 140
all flavors, except chocolate flavors *(Duncan Hines)* 130
all flavors, except chocolate and lemon *(Betty Crocker
    Whipped Deluxe)* 100
banana, lemon, or strawberry creme *(Pillsbury Creamy
    Supreme)* 150
caramel pecan *(Pillsbury Creamy Supreme)* 150
chocolate, all flavors *(Duncan Hines)* 140
chocolate, all flavors, except dark *(Pillsbury Creamy
    Supreme)* 140
chocolate, dark *(Pillsbury Creamy Supreme)* 130
chocolate or lemon *(Betty Crocker Whipped Deluxe)* . . . 110
coconut pecan *(Pillsbury Creamy Supreme)* 160
cream cheese *(Pillsbury Creamy Supreme)* 150
fudge, hot *(Pillsbury Creamy Supreme)* 140
vanilla *(Pillsbury Creamy Supreme)* 150
Frozen desserts, see "Ice cream"
Fruit, see specific listings
Fruit, mixed, candied *(S&W Glace)*, 2 tbsp. 90
Fruit, mixed, canned (see also "Fruit cocktail"),
    ½ cup:
in juice, chunky *(Del Monte)* 60
in juice, chunky *(Libby's Lite)* 60
in extra light syrup, chunky *(Del Monte)* 60
in heavy syrup, chunky *(Del Monte)* 100
salad, tropical, in light syrup *(Del Monte)* 80
salad, tropical, in light syrup *(Dole)* 80
Fruit, mixed, dried:
(Dole Sun Giant), 1.5 oz. 100
(Sonoma), 1.4 oz. 120

Fruit, mixed, dried *(cont.)*
and nuts, see "Trail mix"
Fruit, mixed, frozen *(Stilwell)*, 1 cup 50
Fruit bar, frozen (see also "Ice bar" and "Yogurt bar"),
 1 bar:
all flavors *(Dole* Fruit Juice) 45
all flavors *(Dole* Fruit Juice No Sugar) 25
all flavors *(Dole* Fruit 'n Juice), 2.5 oz. 70
banana cream *(Frozfruit)* 150
cantaloupe *(Frozfruit)* 60
cherry *(Frozfruit)* 70
coconut *(Dole* Fruit 'n Juice), 4 oz. 210
coconut *(Edy's/Dreyer's Grand)* 140
coconut or piña colada cream *(Frozfruit)* 170
lemon, lime, or orange *(Frozfruit)* 90
lemonade *(Dole* Fruit 'n Juice), 4-oz. bar 120
lime or strawberry *(Dole* Fruit 'n Juice), 4-oz. bar 110
lime or strawberry *(Edy's/Dreyer's Grand)* 90
peach *(Edy's/Dreyer's Grand)* 140
pine-coconut *(Dole* Fruit 'n Juice), 4-oz. bar 150
pine-orange-banana *(Dole* Fruit 'n Juice), 4-oz. bar 110
pineapple, raspberry, or strawberry *(Frozfruit)* 80
raspberry-kiwi *(Edy's/Dreyer's Grand)* 90
strawberry banana cream *(Frozfruit)* 140
tropical *(Frozfruit)* 90
Fruit cocktail, canned, ½ cup:
(Del Monte Very Cherry) 90
(Hunt's) 90
in juice *(Libby's* Lite) 60
in juice *(S&W* Natural) 80
in juice or extra light syrup *(Del Monte)* 80
in heavy syrup *(Del Monte)* 100
in heavy syrup *(S&W)* 90
natural honey flavor *(Del Monte)* 80
Fruit drink blends (see also specific listings):
(Dole Fruit Fiesta), 16 fl. oz. 270
(Dole Lanai/Tropical Breeze), 16 fl. oz. 240
all flavors *(Shasta Plus)*, 12 fl. oz. 170
nectar *(Kern's* Tropical), 11.5 fl. oz. 210
punch *(Farmer's Market* Tropical), 8 fl. oz. 120

punch *(Hi-C)*, 8 fl. oz. 110
punch *(Snapple)*, 8 fl. oz. 110
punch *(Tropicana Twister)*, 8 fl. oz. 140
Fruit juice blends (see also specific listings), 8 fl. oz.,
   except as noted:
(Ceres Medley of Fruit) 120
(Dole Fiesta) 140
(R.W. Knudsen Morning Blend/Vita) 120
(R.W. Knudsen Natural Breakfast) 110
punch *(After the Fall* Maui) 90
punch *(After the Fall* Sangria de la Noche) 125
punch *(Dole)*, 10 fl. oz. 160
punch *(Juicy Juice)* 130
punch *(Veryfine* Juice-Ups) 140
tropical *(Juicy Juice)* 130
tropical, chilled or frozen* *(Dole)* 160
frozen* *(R.W. Knudsen* Natural Breakfast) 110
Fruit snack, all flavors:
(Fruit By the Foot), 1 roll 80
(Fruit Roll Ups), 2 rolls 110
(Fruit Roll Ups Pouch), 1 roll 50
(Stretch Island), 1 oz. 90
Fruit spreads (see also "Jam and preserves"), 1 tbsp.:
all varieties *(Kraft* Reduced Calorie) 20
all varieties *(Polaner)* 40
all varieties *(R.W. Knudsen)* 50
Fruit syrup (see also specific listings), 1/4 cup:
(Smucker's) 210
light *(Smucker's)* 130
and maple *(R.W. Knudsen)* 150
Fudge topping, see "Chocolate topping"
Fusilli pasta, refrigerated *(Tutta Pasta)*, 1 cup 290
Fusilli pasta mix, w/creamy pesto *(Knorr)*, 2/3 cup 250

G

Gai lan, see "Kale, Chinese"
Garbanzo beans, see "Chickpeas"
Garlic:
(Frieda's Elephant), 1 tbsp. 5
1 clove, approx. .1 oz. 4
crushed *(Christopher Ranch),* 1 tsp. 10
Garlic dip *(Nalley),* 2 tbsp. 130
Garlic pepper, 1 tsp. 8
Garlic pickle relish *(Patak's),* 1 tbsp. 45
Garlic powder, 1 tsp. 10
Garlic salt, 1 tsp. 3
Garlic spread *(Lawry's* Concentrate), 2 tsp. 50
Garlic sprouts *(Jonathan's),* 1 cup, 4 oz. 70
Garlic and basil, chopped *(Paesana),* 1 tsp. 6
Gelatin, unflavored *(Knox),* 1 pkt. 25
Gelatin dessert, all flavors *(Hunt's Snack Pack),* ½ cup . 100
Gelatin dessert mix*:
all flavors *(Jell-O),* ½ cup 80
all flavors *(Jell-O* Sugar Free), ½ cup 10
strawberry *(Jell-O 1-2-3),* ⅔ cup 130
Ghee, see "Butter, clarified"
Ginger, trimmed root, sliced, ¼ cup 17
Ginger, ground, 1 tsp. 6
Ginger, pickled *(Eden),* 1 tbsp. 15
Ginger drink *(Santa Cruz* Hawaiian), 8 fl. oz. 110
Ginkgo nut, canned, drained, 1 oz. 32
Glaze, fruit:
for banana, creamy *(Marie's),* 2 tbsp. 60
for blueberries, peaches, or strawberries *(Marie's),*
   2 tbsp. 40
pie, strawberry *(Smucker's),* 2 oz. 80
Glaze mix, see specific listings
Goat, meat only, roasted, 4 oz. 162

Gobo root, see "Burdock root"
Godfather's Pizza, 1 slice:
cheese, original crust:
    mini, 1/4 pie 131
    medium, 1/8 pie 231
    large, 1/10 pie 258
    jumbo, 1/10 pie 382
cheese, golden crust:
    medium, 1/8 pie 212
    large, 1/10 pie 242
combo, original crust:
    mini, 1/4 pie 176
    medium, 1/8 pie 306
    large, 1/10 pie 338
    jumbo, 1/10 pie 503
combo, golden crust:
    medium, 1/8 pie 271
    large, 1/10 pie 305
Golden nugget squash *(Frieda's),* 3/4 cup, 3 oz. 30
Goose, roasted:
meat w/skin, 4 oz. 346
meat only, 4 oz. 270
Goose liver, see "Liver" and "Pâté"
Gooseberry, canned, 1/2 cup:
in light syrup *(Comstock)* 70
in light syrup *(Oregon)* 90
Gorgonzola sauce *(Monterey Pasta Company),* 4 oz. . . . 400
Grains, see specific listings
Granola, see "Cereal"
Grape:
fresh, 10 medium, except as noted:
    (Frieda's), 5 oz. 100
    American type (slipskin) 15
    European type (adherent skin), seedless 36
canned, Thompson seedless:
    in light syrup *(Oregon),* 1/2 cup 100
    in heavy syrup *(S&W),* 1/2 cup 100
    spiced, in heavy syrup *(Oregon),* 1/2 cup 110
Grape drink, 8 fl. oz., except as noted:
(Capri Sun), 6.75 fl. oz. 110

(Dole), 10 fl. oz. 150
(Tropicana Twister) 130
(Veryfine Glacial) 110
grape watermelon squeeze or grapeade *(Snapple)* 110
frozen* *(Minute Maid)* 120
Grape juice, 8 fl. oz.:
(Juicy Juice) 130
(Veryfine) 180
(Veryfine Juice-Ups) 130
bottled or frozen* *(R.W. Knudsen)* 150
Grape leaves, stuffed *(Cedar's)*, 6 pieces, 4.94 oz. 180
Grapefruit, fresh:
pink or red, California or Arizona, ½ medium 46
pink or red, Florida, ½ medium 37
white, California, ½ medium 43
white, Florida, ½ medium 38
Grapefruit, canned or chilled:
(S&W Natural Style), ⅔ cup 50
in juice, pink or white *(Sunfresh)*, ½ cup 45
Grapefruit drink, pink, 8 fl. oz.:
(Tree Top Desert Ice) 120
(Tropicana Twister) 120
(Tropicana Twister Light) 35
Grapefruit juice, 8 fl. oz., except as noted:
fresh, 6 fl. oz. 72
(Dole), 10 fl. oz. 120
(S&W) 100
(Snapple Pink), 12 fl. oz. 190
(Tree Top) 100
(Veryfine) 90
blend *(Dole* Sunripe) 130
blend, cranberry *(Apple & Eve* Ruby Red) 120
golden *(Tropicana)* 90
ruby red *(Tropicana* Carton/Plastic) 100
frozen* *(Minute Maid)* 100
Gravy, see specific listings
Great northern beans, ½ cup:
boiled 104
canned *(Allens)* 100
canned *(Eden* Organic Jars) 120

Great northern beans *(cont.)*
canned *(Stokely)* 110
canned, w/sausage *(Trappey's)* 100
Green beans, fresh:
raw *(Dole)*, ¾ cup, 3 oz. 25
boiled, drained, ½ cup 22
Green beans, canned, ½ cup:
(Stokely/Stokely No Salt) 20
all varieties *(Seneca)* 25
all varieties, except Italian cut *(Del Monte)* 20
all varieties, except whole *(Green Giant)* 20
whole *(Green Giant)* 25
whole, cut, or French style *(S&W)* 20
cut *(Allens/Sunshine/Alma/Crest Top)* 30
cut *(Green Giant/Green Giant* Less Sodium) 20
cut, w/wax beans *(S&W)* 20
French style *(Green Giant)* 20
Italian *(Allens)* 30
Italian cut *(Del Monte)* 30
and potatoes *(Allens/Sunshine)* 35
Green beans, dilled *(S&W)*, 1 oz. 20
Green beans, frozen:
(Seabrook), 1 cup 25
(Seneca), ¾ cup 30
cut *(Green Giant)*, ¾ cup 25
sliced *(Stilwell)*, ⅔ cup 25
Green bean combinations, frozen:
mushroom casserole *(Stouffer's)*, 3.8 oz. 140
w/toasted almonds *(Birds Eye)*, ¾ cup 80
Green peas, see "Peas, green"
Greens, mixed, canned *(Allens/Sunshine)*, ½ cup 30
Grenadine syrup *(Rose's)*, 2 tbsp. 90
Grilling sauce (see also specific listings):
Chardonnay or Tuscan herb *(Knorr)*, 2 tbsp. 35
mandarin ginger *(Knorr* Microwave), 2 tbsp. 45
Parmesano *(Knorr* Microwave), 3 tbsp. 50
plum, spicy *(Knorr)*, 2 tbsp. 50
tequila lime *(Knorr)*, 2 tbsp. 40
Grits, see "Corn grits"
Grouper, meat only, baked or broiled, 4 oz. 134

Guacamole, see "Avocado dip"

Guanabana, frozen, chunks *(Goya),* ⅓ pkg. 60

Guava, 1 medium, 4 oz. 45

Guava drink *(Snapple* Guava Mania), 8 fl. oz. 110

Guava juice *(After the Fall* Maya), 8 fl. oz. 110

Guava nectar *(Kern's),* 8 fl. oz. 150

Guinea hen, raw:

meat w/skin, 4 oz. 179

meat only, 4 oz. 125

Gumbo dinner mix *(Luzianne),* ⅕ pkg. 160

Gyro mix *(Casbah),* ¹⁄₁₀ pkg. 64

H

FOOD AND MEASURE   **CALORIES**

Häagen-Dazs Ice Cream Shop:
ice cream, ½ cup:
    butter pecan 320
    Brownies à la Mode (Exträas) 280
    Cappuccino Commotion (Exträas) 310
    Caramel Cone Explosion (Exträas) 310
    chocolate 270
    chocolate almond, Swiss 300
    chocolate chocolate, Belgian 330
    chocolate chocolate chip or mint 300
    chocolate peanut butter, deep 370
    coffee or cookies and cream 270
    coffee chip 290
    Cookie Dough Dynamo (Exträas) 300
    macadamia brittle 300
    macadamia nut 320
    Midnight Cookies and Cream 300
    pralines and cream 290
    rum raisin or vanilla 270
    strawberry 250
    Strawberry Cheesecake Craze (Exträas) 280
    vanilla chocolate chip or vanilla fudge 290
    vanilla Swiss almond 310
ice cream bar, chocolate, uncoated, 1 bar 200
ice cream bar, coffee or vanilla, uncoated, 1 bar 190
sorbet, ½ cup:
    banana strawberry or orchard peach 140
    chocolate or strawberry 130
    mango, raspberry, or *Zesty Lemon* 120
sorbet, soft serve, mango or raspberry, ½ cup 100
yogurt, soft serve, ½ cup:
    chocolate or vanilla, nonfat 110
    chocolate mousse, nonfat 80

Häagen-Dazs, yogurt *(cont.)*
coffee 140
vanilla mousse, nonfat 70
Haddock, meat only:
baked, broiled, or microwaved, 4 oz. 127
smoked (finnan haddie), 4 oz. 132
Haddock entree, frozen:
battered *(Van de Kamp's)*, 2 pieces 260
breaded *(Mrs. Paul's* Premium), 1 piece 230
breaded *(Van de Kamp's)*, 2 pieces 280
breaded *(Van de Kamp's* Light), 1 piece 220
Hake, fresh, see "Whiting"
Halibut, meat only, 4 oz.:
Atlantic and Pacific, baked or broiled 159
Greenland, baked or broiled 271
Halibut, frozen *(Peter Pan)*, 4 oz. 110
Halvah, chocolate *(Joyva)*, 1.75 oz. 340
Ham, fresh, meat only, 4 oz.:
whole leg, roasted, lean w/fat 333
whole leg, roasted, lean only 249
rump half, roasted, lean w/fat 311
rump half, roasted, lean only 251
shank half, roasted, lean w/fat 344
shank half, roasted, lean only 244
Ham, cured, meat only, 4 oz.:
whole leg, lean w/fat, unheated 279
whole leg, roasted 276
whole leg, lean only, unheated 167
whole leg, roasted 178
boneless (11% fat), unheated 206
boneless (11% fat), roasted 202
boneless, extra lean (5% fat), unheated 149
boneless, extra lean (5% fat), roasted 164
Ham, canned or refrigerated, 3 oz.:
(Hormel Light & Lean) 90
(John Morrell Boneless) 140
(Jones Dairy Farm Homestead) 140
Black Forest or maple *(Boar's Head* Baby) 90
honey *(Patrick Cudahy ReaLean)* 90
semi-boneless *(Jones Dairy Farm)* 180

skinless, shankless *(Jones Dairy Farm)* 160
slice, smoked or maple glaze *(Boar's Head Sweet Slice)* . 110
smoke flavor *(Patrick Cudahy ReaLean)* 80
smoked, semi-boneless *(Boar's Head)* 130
spiral sliced *(Spiral Cure 81 Half)* 150
steak, honey *(Patrick Cudahy)* 100
steak, smoke flavor *(Patrick Cudahy)* 90
Virginia *(Boar's Head Ready-to-Eat)* 100
Virginia, smoked *(Boar's Head Baby Gourmet)* 90
"Ham," vegetarian, frozen *(Worthington Wham)*,
   2 slices 80
Ham entree, frozen, steak, w/macaroni and cheese
   (Marie Callender), 14 oz. 490
Ham glaze *(Crosse & Blackwell),* 1 tbsp. 30
Ham lunch meat, 2 oz., except as noted:
(Black Bear Lower Sodium) 50
(Boar's Head Deluxe) 60
(Boar's Head Lower Sodium Extra Lean) 50
(Jones Dairy Farm Lean Choice), 2 slices 50
(Menumaster), 1 oz. 30
(Old Tyme), 1 oz. 35
(Oscar Mayer Lower Sodium), 3 slices 70
all varieties *(Healthy Choice)* 60
baked *(Louis Rich Carving Board),* 2 slices 50
baked *(Oscar Mayer),* 3 slices, 2.2 oz. 70
Black Forest *(Boar's Head)* 60
boiled *(Oscar Mayer),* 3 slices, 2.2 oz. 60
boiled *(Patrick Cudahy),* 1-oz. slice 30
cappacola *(Boar's Head Cappy)* 60
cappacola *(Healthy Deli Cappi)* 60
chopped *(Black Label)* 140
cooked *(Patrick Cudahy Less Sodium),* 1-oz. slice 30
honey *(Healthy Deli Honey Valley Farms)* 60
honey *(Oscar Mayer),* 3 slices, 2.2 oz. 70
honey *(Oscar Mayer Deli-Thin),* 4 slices 60
honey *(Patrick Cudahy),* 1-oz. slice 35
hot, jalapeño, or pepper *(Healthy Deli)* 60
maple *(Boar's Head Honey Coat)* 60
maple glazed *(Black Bear Old Fashioned)* 60
pepper *(Boar's Head)* 70

Ham lunch meat *(cont.)*

smoked *(Boar's Head* Gourmet) 60
smoked *(Louis Rich Carving Board)*, 2 slices 45
spiced *(Boar's Head)* 120
Virginia *(Black Bear)* 50
Virginia *(Boar's Head)* 60
Virginia, baked *(Healthy Deli* Less Sodium) 70

Ham spread:

deviled *(Cure 81)*, 2 oz. 150
deviled *(Underwood)*, 1/4 cup 160
deviled, w/crackers *(Red Devil* Snackers), 1 pkg. 310
honey *(Underwood)*, 1/4 cup 190
honey, w/crackers *(Red Devil* Snackers), 1 pkg. 340
salad *(Libby's Spreadables)*, 1/3 cup 110

Ham and cheese sandwich, frozen, 1 piece:

(Croissant Pockets) 360
(Healthy Choice Hearty Handfuls) 320
(Hormel Quick Meal) 330
(Hot Pockets) 340
(Totino's Big & Hearty) 310

Hamburger, see "Beef sandwich"

"Hamburger," vegetarian, 1 patty, except as noted:

(NewMenu VegiBurger), 3 oz. 110

frozen:

   (Amy's California) 100
   (Amy's Chicago) 160
   (Ken & Robert's Veggie Burger) 110
   (Morningstar Farms Prime Patties) 110
   (Morningstar Farms Better'n Burger) 70
   (Morningstar Farms Grillers) 140
   (Natural Touch Vegan Burger) 70
   all varieties *(Green Giant Harvest Burgers)* 140
   black bean, spicy *(Natural Touch)* 100
   garden grille *(Morningstar Farms)* 120
   garden vegetable *(Morningstar Farms)* 110
   garden vegetable *(Natural Touch)* 110
   tofu *(Natural Touch* Okara) 110

refrigerated *(Hempeh Burger)* 140
refrigerated *(Morningstar Farms* Garden Veggie) 150

"Hamburger," vegetarian, mix:
(Loma Linda Vita Burger Chunks), ¼ cup mix* 70
(Loma Linda Vita Burger Granules), 3 tbsp. mix* 70
(Morningstar Farms Garden Grille Kit), ¼ pkg. 80
(Morningstar Farms Southwestern Kit), ¼ pkg. 90
(Natural Touch Burger Kit), ¼ pkg. 90
(Natural Touch Original Veggie Burger Kit), ¼ pkg. 80
Hamburger entree mix*, 1 cup, except as noted:
beef, barbecue *(Hamburger Helper* BBQ) 320
beef pasta *(Hamburger Helper)* 270
beef Romanoff *(Hamburger Helper)* 280
beef stew *(Hamburger Helper Homestyle)* 250
beef taco *(Hamburger Helper)* 310
beef teriyaki *(Hamburger Helper)* 290
cheddar and bacon *(Hamburger Helper)* 350
cheddar melt *(Hamburger Helper)* 310
cheese, three *(Hamburger Helper)* 340
cheeseburger macaroni *(Hamburger Helper)* 360
chili macaroni *(Hamburger Helper)* 290
fettuccine Alfredo *(Hamburger Helper)* 310
Italian, cheesy *(Hamburger Helper)* 330
Italian, zesty *(Hamburger Helper)* 320
lasagna or Italian rigatoni *(Hamburger Helper)* 280
meat loaf *(Hamburger Helper)*, ⅙ loaf 270
Mexican, zesty *(Hamburger Helper)* 300
mushroom and wild rice *(Hamburger Helper)* 310
nacho cheese *(Hamburger Helper)* 320
pizza *(Hamburger Helper Pizzabake)*, ⅙ pan 270
pizza pasta or potato au gratin *(Hamburger Helper)* 290
potato Stroganoff *(Hamburger Helper)* 270
ravioli *(Hamburger Helper)* 280
rice Oriental *(Hamburger Helper)* 310
Salisbury *(Hamburger Helper)* 270
shells, cheesy *(Hamburger Helper)* 340
spaghetti *(Hamburger Helper)* 300
Stroganoff *(Hamburger Helper)* 320
Swedish meatball *(Hamburger Helper Homestyle)* 300
Hardee's, 1 serving:
breakfast items:
    Big Country Breakfast, bacon 820

Hardee's, breakfast items *(cont.)*

Big Country Breakfast, sausage 1,000

biscuit:

    Apple Cinnamon 'N' Raisin 200

    bacon and egg 570

    bacon, egg, and cheese 610

    country ham 430

    ham 400

    ham, egg, and cheese 540

    jelly 440

    Rise 'N' Shine 390

    sausage 510

    sausage and egg 630

    Ultimate Omelet 570

Biscuit 'N' Gravy 510

Frisco Breakfast Sandwich, ham 500

Hash Rounds, regular 230

pancakes, 3 cakes 280

burgers and sandwiches:

Big Roast Beef sandwich 460

The Boss 570

cheeseburger 310

cheeseburger, mesquite bacon 370

cheeseburger, quarter pound double 470

chicken fillet sandwich 480

Cravin' Bacon cheeseburger 690

Fisherman's Fillet 560

Frisco burger 720

grilled chicken sandwich 350

hamburger 270

hamburger, the works 530

Hot Ham 'N' Cheese 310

Mushroom 'N' Swiss burger 490

roast beef sandwich, regular 320

fried chicken:

breast 370

leg 170

thigh 330

wing 200

sides:
  baked beans, 5 oz. 170
  coleslaw, 4 oz. 240
  fries, small 240
  fries, medium 350
  fries, large 430
  gravy, 1.5 oz. 20
  mashed potato, 4 oz. 70
salads:
  garden 220
  grilled chicken 150
  side salad 25
dressings:
  French, fat free 70
  ranch 290
  Thousand Island 250
desserts and shakes:
  Big Cookie 280
  cone, chocolate 180
  cone, *Cool Twist,* vanilla/chocolate 180
  cone, vanilla 170
  peach cobbler, 6 oz. 310
  shake, chocolate 370
  shake, peach 350
  shake, strawberry 420
  shake, vanilla 350
  sundae, hot fudge 290
  sundae, strawberry 210
Head cheese *(Oscar Mayer),* 1-oz. slice 50
Herbs, see specific listings
Herring, meat only, 4 oz.:
Atlantic, baked or broiled 230
Atlantic, kippered 246
Atlantic, pickled 297
Pacific, baked or broiled 284
Herring, canned, see "Sardine"
Herring, in jars *(Vita* Party Snacks), 2 oz. 120
Herring salad *(Vita),* 1/4 cup 110
Hoisin sauce:
(Ka•Me), 2 tbsp. 45

Hoisin sauce *(cont.)*
(Lee Kum Kee), 2 tbsp. 100
Hollandaise sauce mix *(Knorr)*, ¹/₁₀ pkg. 10
Hominy (see also "Corn grits"), canned, ½ cup:
golden *(Allens/Uncle William)* 120
golden or white *(Van Camp's)* 80
white *(Allens/Uncle William)* 100
white *(Goya)* 100
Honey *(Aunt Sue's/Grandma's/Sue Bee)*, 1 tbsp. 60
Honey loaf *(Oscar Mayer)*, 1-oz. slice 35
Honey roll sausage, beef, 1 oz. 52
Honeydew melon:
(Dole), ¹/₁₀ melon, 4.8 oz. 50
pulp, cubed, ½ cup 30
Horned melon *(Frieda's)*, 3.5-oz. melon 25
Horseradish, prepared:
(Boar's Head), 1 tsp. 0
red *(Rosoff)*, 1 tbsp. 8
white *(Rosoff)*, 1 tbsp. 7
Horseradish sauce:
(Bookbinder's Hot), 1 tsp. 15
(Heinz), 1 tsp. 25
Hot dog, see "Frankfurter"
Hot dog sauce, see "Chili sauce"
Hot fudge sauce, see "Chocolate topping"
Hot sauce, see "Pepper sauce" and specific listings
Hubbard squash:
(Frieda's), ³/₄ cup, 3 oz. 35
boiled, drained, mashed, ½ cup 35
Hummus *(Casbah)*, 1 oz. 85
Hummus dip *(Cedar's* Sports), 2 tbsp. 34
Hummus mix *(Casbah)*, 1 oz. 120
Hush puppies:
frozen *(Stilwell)*, 3 pieces 140
mix *(Martha White)*, ¹/₄ cup fried 300
Hyacinth beans, fresh, boiled, drained, ½ cup 22

FOOD AND MEASURE   **CALORIES**

Ice, Italian, 6 fl. oz.:
cherry *(Luigi's)*	120
chocolate fudge *(Luigi's)*	150
grape, lemon, or strawberry *(Luigi's)*	110

Ice bar (see also "Fruit bar, frozen"), 1 bar:
(Cool Creations Ice Pop)	50
cappuccino *(Frozfruit)*	140
lemon *(Great White)*	70

Ice cream, ½ cup:
almond, praline *(Edy's/Dreyer's Grand)*	170
almond, toasted *(Dreyer's Grand)*	150
amaretto *(Häagen-Dazs DiSaronno)*	260
banana chocolate chunk *(Healthy Choice* Low Fat)	120
banana cream pie *(Edy's Homemade)*	140
banana split *(Edy's Grand)*	160
(Ben & Jerry's Chubby Hubby)	350
(Ben & Jerry's Chunky Monkey)	300
(Ben & Jerry's Cool Britannia)	260
(Ben & Jerry's Holy Cannoli)	270
(Ben & Jerry's Phish Food)	310
(Ben & Jerry's Rainforest Crunch)	300
(Ben & Jerry's Wavy Gravy)	330
Black Forest *(Healthy Choice* Low Fat)	120
brownie, blond, sundae *(Ben & Jerry's* Low Fat)	190
brownie, double fudge *(Edy's Grand)*	170
brownie, double fudge *(Edy's/Dreyer's* No Sugar)	100
brownie, fudge, chocolate *(Ben & Jerry's)*	250
butter pecan *(Ben & Jerry's)*	310
butter pecan *(Edy's/Dreyer's Grand)*	160
butter pecan *(Edy's/Dreyer's Grand* Light)	120
butter pecan *(Edy's/Dreyer's* No Sugar)	110
butter pecan *(Edy's Homemade)*	170
butter pecan *(Häagen-Dazs)*	320

Ice cream *(cont.)*

butter pecan *(Sealtest)*	160
butter pecan crunch *(Healthy Choice Low Fat)*	120
Butterfinger Blast *(Edy's/Dreyer's Grand)*	160
cappuccino chocolate chunk or mocha fudge *(Healthy Choice Low Fat)*	120
caramel cream, dreamy *(Edy's Grand Light)*	110
caramel praline crunch *(Edy's/Dreyer's Fat Free)*	120
cherry chocolate chip *(Ben & Jerry's Cherry Garcia)*	240
cherry chocolate or espresso chip *(Edy's Grand)*	150
cherry chocolate chunk *(Edy's/Dreyer's Grand)*	150
cherry chocolate chunk *(Healthy Choice Low Fat)*	110
cherry vanilla *(Breyers All Natural)*	150
cherry vanilla, black, swirl *(Edy's Fat Free)*	100
cherry vanilla, black, swirl *(Edy's/Dreyer's No Sugar)*	90
Chiquita 'N chocolate *(Edy's/Dreyer's Grand Light)*	110
chocolate *(Edy's/Dreyer's Grand)*	220
chocolate *(Häagen-Dazs)*	270
chocolate *(Sealtest)*	140
chocolate, triple *(Edy's/Dreyer's No Sugar)*	100
chocolate almond fudge *(Edy's/Dreyer's Grand Light)*	120
chocolate brownie chunk *(Edy's/Dreyer's Fat Free)*	120
chocolate chip *(Edy's/Dreyer's Grand Chips!)*	170
chocolate chip *(Edy's Homemade)*	180
chocolate chip *(Sealtest)*	150
chocolate chip, chocolate *(Häagen-Dazs)*	300
chocolate chip, mint *(Breyers All Natural)*	170
chocolate chip, mint *(Edy's/Dreyer's Grand Chips!)*	170
chocolate chip, mint *(Sealtest)*	150
chocolate chip cookie dough *(Ben & Jerry's)*	270
chocolate chip cookie dough *(Sealtest)*	160
chocolate chocolate chunk *(Healthy Choice Low Fat)*	120
chocolate chunk, double *(Edy's Homemade)*	190
chocolate cookie, mint *(Ben & Jerry's)*	260
chocolate fudge *(Edy's/Dreyer's Fat Free)*	120
chocolate fudge *(Edy's/Dreyer's Fat Free/No Sugar)*	100
chocolate fudge mousse *(Edy's Grand)*	160
chocolate fudge mousse *(Edy's/Dreyer's Grand Light)*	110
chocolate fudge mousse *(Healthy Choice Low Fat)*	120
chocolate fudge sundae *(Edy's Grand)*	170

chocolate mumbo jumbo *(Edy's/Dreyer's Grand)* 170
chocolate peanut butter chunk *(Edy's/Dreyer's Fat Free)* . 120
coffee *(Ben & Jerry's Coffee Coffee Buzz Buzz Buzz)* . . . 290
coffee *(Breyers All Natural)* 150
coffee *(Edy's/Dreyer's Grand)* 140
coffee, Italian roast *(Starbuck's)* 230
coffee, latte *(Starbuck's Low Fat)* 170
coffee or cookies and cream *(Häagen-Dazs)* 270
coffee and biscotti *(Ben & Jerry's Low Fat)* 170
coffee fudge *(Edy's/Dreyer's Fat Free)* 110
coffee fudge *(Edy's/Dreyer's Fat Free/No Sugar)* 100
coffee fudge *(Häagen-Dazs Fat Free)* 170
coffee java chip *(Starbuck's)* 250
coffee toffee crunch *(Ben & Jerry's Heath)* 280
cookie chunk *(Edy's/Dreyer's Fat Free)* 120
cookie creme de mint *(Healthy Choice Low Fat)* 130
cookie dough *(Edy's/Dreyer's Grand)* 170
cookie dough *(Edy's/Dreyer's Grand Light)* 130
cookies 'n cream *(Edy's/Dreyer's Grand)* 160
cookies 'n cream *(Edy's/Dreyer's Grand Light)* 110
cookies 'n cream *(Healthy Choice Low Fat)* 120
cookies 'n cream mint *(Dreyer's Grand Light)* 110
cream, sweet, and cookies *(Ben & Jerry's Low Fat)* 170
espresso fudge chip *(Dreyer's Grand Light)* 120
French silk *(Edy's/Dreyer's Grand Light)* 120
fudge, marble *(Edy's/Dreyer's Fat Free)* 110
fudge, marble *(Edy's/Dreyer's No Sugar)* 90
fudge, mint *(Dreyer's Fat Free)* 110
fudge brownie *(Healthy Choice Low Fat)* 120
fudge chunk *(Ben & Jerry's New York)* 290
fudge royal or heavenly hash *(Sealtest)* 150
ice cream sandwich *(Edy's Grand)* 140
Irish cream *(Häagen-Dazs Baileys)* 270
macadamia brittle *(Häagen-Dazs)* 300
mint chocolate chip *(Healthy Choice Low Fat)* 120
mocha *(Starbuck's Low Fat Mambo)* 170
mocha fudge *(Edy's/Dreyer's No Sugar)* 90
mocha fudge almond *(Dreyer's Grand)* 170
mocha fudge almond *(Dreyer's Grand Light)* 120
mud pie *(Dreyer's Grand)* 160

Ice cream *(cont.)*

Neapolitan *(Dreyer's Grand)*	140
peach *(Breyers All Natural)*	130
peanut butter cup *(Ben & Jerry's)*	370
peanut butter cup *(Edy's Grand Light Cups!)*	130
praline and caramel *(Healthy Choice Low Fat)*	130
praline caramel cluster *(Healthy Choice Low Fat)*	130
raspberry ribbon, wild *(Healthy Choice Low Fat)*	110
raspberry vanilla swirl *(Edy's/Dreyer's Fat Free/No Sugar)*	90
rocky road *(Edy's/Dreyer's Grand)*	170
rocky road *(Edy's/Dreyer's Grand Light)*	110
rocky road *(Healthy Choice Low Fat)*	140
rum raisin *(Häagen-Dazs)*	270
(Starbuck's Biscotti Bliss)	230
strawberry *(Edy's/Dreyer's Grand Real)*	130
strawberry *(Edy's/Dreyer's No Sugar)*	80
strawberry *(Häagen-Dazs)*	250
strawberry *(Häagen-Dazs Fat Free)*	150
strawberry *(Sealtest)*	130
strawberries and cream *(Edy's Homemade)*	140
turtle fudge cake *(Healthy Choice Low Fat)*	130
vanilla *(Ben & Jerry's)*	250
vanilla *(Edy's/Dreyer's Fat Free/Edy's/Dreyer's Grand Light)*	100
vanilla *(Edy's/Dreyer's No Sugar)*	80
vanilla *(Edy's/Dreyer's Fat Free/No Sugar)*	90
vanilla *(Edy's Homemade)*	160
vanilla *(Edy's/Dreyer's Grand)*	150
vanilla *(Edy's/Dreyer's Grand Avalanche)*	170
vanilla *(Häagen-Dazs)*	270
vanilla *(Healthy Choice Low Fat)*	100
vanilla *(Sealtest)*	140
vanilla, French *(Edy's/Dreyer's Grand)*	160
vanilla, French *(Sealtest)*	140
vanilla bean *(Edy's/Dreyer's Grand)*	130
vanilla caramel fudge swirl *(Ben & Jerry's)*	280
vanilla 'n caramel *(Edy's/Dreyer's Fat Free/No Sugar)*	100
vanilla 'n caramel *(Edy's/Dreyer's No Sugar)*	90
vanilla and chocolate *(Edy's Grand)*	150

vanilla-chocolate mint patty *(Ben & Jerry's* Low Fat) . . . 180
vanilla-chocolate-strawberry *(Breyers* All Natural) 150
vanilla-chocolate-strawberry *(Edy's Grand)* 140
vanilla-chocolate-strawberry *(Sealtest)* 140
vanilla chocolate swirl *(Edy's/Dreyer's* Fat Free/No
  Sugar) 90
vanilla fudge *(Häagen-Dazs)* 280
vanilla fudge twirl *(Breyers* All Natural) 160
vanilla mocha swirl *(Starbuck's)* 270
vanilla Swiss almond *(Häagen-Dazs)* 310
vanilla w/toffee crunch *(Ben & Jerry's* Heath) 280
"Ice cream," nondairy, ½ cup, except as noted:
all flavors *(Tofutti* Soft Serve) 190
all flavors *(Tofutti* Soft Serve Lite) 90
all fruit flavors *(Tofutti Fruitti)* 100
chocolate *(Tofutti)* 180
chocolate cake *(Tofutti)* 210
chocolate fudge *(Tofutti* Low Fat) 120
coffee marshmallow *(Tofutti* Low Fat) 100
peach mango or strawberry banana *(Tofutti* Low Fat) . . . 100
pecan, better *(Tofutti)* 220
stick, chocolate *(Tofutti Fruitti),* 1 piece 120
stick, fudge *(Tofutti* Teddy), 1 piece 70
stick, fudge *(Tofutti* Treats), 1 piece 30
vanilla or vanilla fudge *(Tofutti)* 190
vanilla almond bark *(Tofutti)* 210
vanilla fudge *(Tofutti* Low Fat) 120
wildberry *(Tofutti)* 190
wildberry, chocolate covered *(Tofutti* Slice), 1 slice 180
Ice cream bar, 1 bar, except as noted:
almond *(DoveBar* Singles), 3.5 oz. 350
almond *(Klondike)* 310
(Ben & Jerry's Chunky Monkey) 360
(Butterfinger) 190
caramel creme swirl w/toffee chips *(DoveBar)* 280
cherry royale *(Dove Bite Size),* 5 bars 340
chocolate *(Fudgsicle* Bar), 2.5 oz. or 2.7 oz. 90
chocolate *(Nestlé Crunch)* 200
chocolate, w/dark chocolate *(DoveBar* Single), 3.5 oz. . . 330

Ice cream bar *(cont.)*

chocolate, w/dark chocolate *(Häagen-Dazs* Single),
    4 oz. 400
chocolate, double *(Dove Bite Size),* 5 bars 330
chocolate, w/milk chocolate *(Milky Way)* 220
chocolate cookie dough *(Ben & Jerry's)* 420
coffee almond crunch *(Häagen-Dazs* Single), 3.7 oz. . . . 360
cookies 'n cream *(Edy's/Dreyer's)* 250
mocha cashew crunch *(DoveBar)* 260
(Nestlé Crunch Crunch King) 270
peanut butter *(Reese's NutRageous)* 240
(Snickers Singles) 200
(Snickers Snack Size), 4 bars 390
vanilla *(Ben & Jerry's)* 330
vanilla *(Good Humor),* 2.75 oz. 180
vanilla *(Klondike* Original) 290
vanilla *(Nestlé Crunch)* 200
vanilla, French *(Dove Bite Size),* 5 bars 330
vanilla, w/almonds *(Edy's/Dreyer's)* 270
vanilla, w/almonds *(Häagen-Dazs* Single), 3.7 oz. 370
vanilla, w/dark chocolate *(DoveBar* Single), 3.5 oz. 330
vanilla, w/dark chocolate *(Häagen-Dazs* Single), 4 oz. . . . 390
vanilla, w/dark chocolate *(Klondike)* 290
vanilla, w/dark chocolate *(Milky Way)* 220
vanilla, ice coated *(Creamsicle* Bar), 2.7 oz. 110
vanilla, w/milk chocolate *(DoveBar* Single), 3.5 oz. 330
vanilla, w/milk chocolate *(Edy's/Dreyer's)* 250
vanilla, w/milk chocolate *(Häagen-Dazs* Single), 3.5 oz. . 330
vanilla, w/toffee crunch *(Ben & Jerry's Heath)* 330
vanilla, white coated *(DoveBar)* 270
vanilla brownie *(Ben & Jerry's)* 330
Ice cream cone, filled, 1 cone:
butter pecan *(Breyers)* 300
chocolate *(Drumstick)* 320
chocolate dipped *(Drumstick)* 320
chocolate dipped *(Good Humor* Premium Sundae) 290
chocolate dipped, w/peanuts *(Good Humor* King) 300
chocolate dipped, w/peanuts *(Klondike* Sundae) 310
cookies 'n cream *(Edy's/Dreyer's* Sundae) 250
(Snickers) 290

vanilla *(Drumstick)* 340
vanilla caramel *(Drumstick)* 360
vanilla fudge *(Drumstick)* 360
vanilla fudge *(Edy's/Dreyer's* Sundae) 240
vanilla fudge ripple *(Good Humor* Choco Taco) 310
Ice cream loaf, all flavors *(Vienetta),* 2.4-oz. slice 190
Ice cream nuggets, chocolate coated:
(Nestlé Crunch), 8 pieces 310
dark *(Bon-Bons),* 8 pieces 310
milk *(Bon-Bons),* 8 pieces 330
Ice cream sandwich, 1 piece:
(Good Humor American Glory), 3.5 oz. 190
(Good Humor Giant), 5 oz. 240
(Häagen-Dazs) 260
(Klondike Big Bear), 5 oz. 200
chocolate chip cookie *(Chipwich* Jr.) 240
chocolate chip cookie *(Good Humor* Premium) 290
Ice cream and sorbet, see "Sorbet"
Icing, see "Frosting"
Italian sausage, see "Sausage" and "Turkey sausage"

FOOD AND MEASURE   **CALORIES**

Jack-in-the-Box, 1 serving:
breakfast:

Breakfast Jack	300
Country Crock Spread, .2 oz.	25
croissant, sausage	670
croissant, supreme	570
hash browns	160
jelly, grape, .5 oz.	40
pancake platter	400
pancake syrup, 1½ oz.	120
sandwich, breakfast, sourdough	380
sandwich, breakfast, ultimate	620
scrambled egg pocket	430

sandwiches:

cheeseburger, regular	320
cheeseburger, double	450
cheeseburger, ultimate	1,030
chicken	400
chicken, Caesar	520
chicken, spicy crispy	560
chicken, supreme	620
chicken fajita pita	290
chicken fillet, grilled	430
hamburger, regular	280
hamburger, quarter-pounder	510
hamburger, sourdough, grilled	670
Jumbo Jack	560
Jumbo Jack w/cheese	650

entrees:

chicken teriyaki bowl	580
taco	190
taco, monster	283
salad, chicken, garden	200

Jack-in-the-Box (cont.)

salad, side 70

finger foods:

    chicken strips, 4 290

    chicken strips, 6 450

    egg rolls, 3 440

    egg rolls, 5 750

    jalapeños, stuffed, 7 420

    jalapeños, stuffed, 10 600

    potato wedges w/bacon, cheddar 800

side dishes:

    fries, small 220

    fries, regular 350

    fries, jumbo 400

    fries, super scoop 590

    fries, seasoned, curly 360

    onion rings 380

sauces:

    barbeque, 1 oz. 45

    buttermilk, .9 oz. 130

    soy, .3 oz. 5

    sweet and sour, 1 oz. 40

    tartar, 1 oz. 150

dressings, 2 oz.:

    blue cheese 210

    buttermilk, house 290

    Italian, low calorie 25

    Thousand Island 250

condiments:

    cheese, American, 1 slice 45

    cheese, Swiss-style, 1 slice 40

    croutons, .4 oz. 50

    hot sauce or mustard pkt. 5

    ketchup pkt. 10

    mayonnaise pkt. 150

    salsa, 1 oz. 10

desserts:

    apple turnover 350

    carrot cake 370

    cheesecake 310

cheesecake, chocolate chip cookie dough 360
shakes:
chocolate or cappuccino 630
strawberry 640
vanilla 610
Jackfruit *(Frieda's),* ⅓ cup, 1.4 oz. 120
Jackson wonder beans *(Frieda's),* ½ cup, 1.2 oz. 120
Jalapeño, see "Pepper, jalapeño"
Jalapeño dip, 2 tbsp.:
(Old El Paso) 30
and cheddar *(Breakstone's)* 60
Jalapeño relish *(Old El Paso),* 1 tbsp. 5
Jam and preserves (see also "Fruit spreads"), 1 tbsp.:
all varieties *(Smucker's)* 50
all varieties *(Smucker's* Light) 10
all varieties *(Smucker's* Reduced Sugar) 25
Jambalaya dinner mix *(Luzianne),* ¼ pkg. 200
Java plum, 3 medium, .4 oz. 5
Jelly, 1 tbsp.:
all fruit flavors *(Smucker's)* 50
apple mint *(Crosse & Blackwell)* 50
currant, red *(Crosse & Blackwell)* 60
grape *(Goya)* 45
guava *(Goya)* 50
pepper, mild *(Tabasco)* 60
pepper, spicy *(Tabasco)* 50
Jerk sauce *(World Harbors* Blue Mountain), 2 tbsp. 80
Jerusalem artichoke *(Frieda's Sun Choke),* ½ cup,
3 oz. 70
Jicama, see "Yam bean tuber"
Kabocha squash *(Frieda's),* ¾ cup, 3 oz. 30
Kale, ½ cup, except as noted:
fresh, raw, chopped *(Dole)* 17
fresh, boiled, drained, chopped 21
canned *(Allens/Sunshine)* 25
frozen *(Seabrook),* 3 oz. 30
Kale, Chinese *(Frieda's* Gai Lan), 1 cup, 3 oz. 15
Kale, Scotch, boiled, drained, chopped, ½ cup 18
Kasha, see "Buckwheat groats"

Ketchup, 1 tbsp.:
(Del Monte) 15
(Healthy Choice) 10
(Heinz) 15
(Hunt's/Hunt's No Salt) 15
(Smucker's) 25
KFC, 1 serving:
chicken, *Original Recipe:*
    breast 400
    drumstick or whole wing 140
    thigh 250
chicken, *Extra Tasty Crispy:*
    breast 470
    drumstick 190
    thigh 370
    wing, whole 200
chicken, Hot & Spicy:
    breast 530
    drumstick 190
    thigh 370
    wing, whole 210
chicken, *Tender Roast:*
    breast, w/skin 251
    breast, w/out skin 169
    drumstick, w/skin 97
    drumstick, w/out skin 67
    thigh, w/skin 207
    thigh, w/out skin 106
    wing, w/skin 121
chicken potpie 770
Chicken Twister 550
Crispy Strips, Colonel's, 3 pieces 261
Crispy Strips, spicy Buffalo, 3 pieces 350
Hot Wings, 6 pieces 471
sandwich, chicken, BBQ flavored 256
sandwich, chicken, *Original Recipe* 497
sides and specials:
    BBQ baked beans, 5.5 oz. 190
    biscuit, 2-oz. piece 180
    coleslaw, 5 oz. 180

```
corn on the cob, 5.7 oz. . . . . . . . . . . . . . . . . . 150
corn bread, 2-oz. piece . . . . . . . . . . . . . . . . 228
green beans, 4.7 oz. . . . . . . . . . . . . . . . . . . . 45
macaroni and cheese, 5.4 oz. . . . . . . . . . . . . 180
mashed potatoes w/gravy, 4.8 oz. . . . . . . . . . 120
*Mean Greens,* 5.4 oz. . . . . . . . . . . . . . . . . . . 70
potato salad, 5.6 oz. . . . . . . . . . . . . . . . . . . 230
potato wedges, 4.8 oz. . . . . . . . . . . . . . . . . . 280
```

Kidney beans, ½ cup:
dry, boiled 112
canned, red:
   (Eden Organic) 100
   (Progresso) 110
   baked *(B&M/Friends)* 170
   dark *(Allens/East Texas Fair/Trappey)* 130
   dark, red or light *(Van Camp)* 90
   dark or light *(Stokely)* 120
   light *(Allens/Trappey's)* 120
   light, w/bacon, chili gravy, or jalapeños *(Trappey's)* . 110
canned, white *(Progresso* Cannellini) 100
Kielbasa (see also "Polish sausage"):
(Boar's Head), 2 oz. 120
(Jones Dairy Farm Dinner), 1 link 190
Kimchee *(Frieda's),* ¼ cup 15
Kiwi, fresh:
(Frieda's), 5 oz. 90
1 large, 3.7 oz. 55
1 medium, 3.1 oz. 46
Kiwi, dried *(Sonoma),* 7–8 pieces, 1 oz. 90
Kiwi-strawberry drink *(Snapple* Cocktail), 8 fl. oz. 110
Knockwurst, beef *(Boar's Head),* 4 oz. 310
Kohlrabi:
raw *(Frieda's),* ⅔ cup, 3 oz. 25
boiled, drained, sliced, ½ cup 24
Kumquat *(Frieda's),* 5 oz. 90

L

Lamb, choice, meat only, 4 oz.:
cubed, leg/shoulder, braised or stewed 253
cubed, leg/shoulder, broiled 211
ground, broiled 321
leg, whole, roasted, lean w/fat 293
leg, whole, roasted, lean only 217
leg, shank, roasted, lean w/fat 255
leg, shank, roasted, lean only 204
leg, sirloin, roasted, lean w/fat 331
leg, sirloin, roasted, lean only 231
loin, roasted, lean w/fat 350
loin, roasted, lean only 229
loin chop, broiled, lean w/fat 358
loin chop, broiled, lean only 245
rib, broiled, lean w/fat 409
rib, broiled, lean only 266
rib, roasted, lean w/fat 407
rib, roasted, lean only 263
shoulder, whole, braised, lean w/fat 390
shoulder, whole, braised, lean only 321
shoulder, whole, roasted, lean w/fat 313
shoulder, whole, roasted, lean only 231
Lamb, New Zealand, frozen, meat only, 4 oz.:
leg, whole, roasted, lean w/fat 279
leg, whole, roasted, lean only 205
Lard *(Goya),* 1 tbsp. 130
Lasagna entree, canned:
(Hormel), 7½ oz. 250
(Hormel Micro Cup), 7½ oz. 250
(Nalley), 1 cup 250
and beef *(Hormel* Micro Cup), 10½ oz. 359
Italian *(Top Shelf),* 10 oz. 340

Lasagna entree, frozen:
(Celentano), 10 oz. 400
(Healthy Choice Roma), 13.5 oz. 400
bake *(Stouffer's)*, 10¼ oz. 370
cheese *(Lean Cuisine Classic)*, 11.5 oz. 290
cheese, w/chicken scallopini *(Lean Cuisine Cafe
    Classics)*, 10 oz. 290
cheese, five *(Lean Cuisine 96 oz.)*, approx. 1 cup 230
extra cheese *(Marie Callender)*, 1 cup, 7.5 oz. 350
Florentine *(Smart Ones)*, 10 oz. 200
garden *(Weight Watchers)*, 11 oz. 270
w/meat sauce:
    (Banquet), 9.5 oz. 260
    (Banquet Family Size), 1 cup, 8 oz. 300
    (Freezer Queen Deluxe Family), 1 cup, 8.3 oz. 270
    (Lean Cuisine), 10.5 oz. 290
    (Marie Callender), 1 cup, 7.5 oz. 370
    (Stouffer's), 10.5 oz. 370
    casserole *(Swanson Lunch and More)*, 1 pkg. 340
primavera *(Celentano Great Choice)*, 10 oz. 240
vegetable *(Lean Cuisine)*, 10.5 oz. 270
vegetable, w/cheese *(Amy's)*, 9.5 oz. 300
vegetable, cheesy, casserole *(Swanson Lunch and
    More)*, 1 pkg. 350
zucchini *(Healthy Choice)*, 13.5 oz. 280
Leek, fresh:
raw *(Frieda's)*, 1 cup, 3 oz. 50
raw, 9.9-oz. leek 76
boiled, drained, chopped, ½ cup 16
Lemon *(Dole)*, 1 lemon 18
Lemon herb sauce mix *(Knorr)*, 1 tbsp. 30
Lemon juice, fresh, 1 tbsp. 4
Lemon peel, candied *(S&W)*, 1.1 oz. 80
Lemon pepper, 1 tsp. 7
Lemon sauce (see also "Stir-fry sauce"):
(House of Tsang), 2 tbsp. 70
(Ka•Me), 1 tbsp. 45
pepper garlic *(World Harbors)*, 2 tbsp. 35
Lemonade, 8 fl. oz., except as noted:
(After the Fall) 90

(Heinke's Old Fashion) 120
(Minute Maid) 110
(Santa Cruz) 120
(Snapple) 100
(Veryfine Chillers), 11.5 fl. oz. 180
pink *(Snapple* Diet) 20
pink *(Tropicana Twister)* 120
pink *(Veryfine* Chillers), 11.5 fl. oz. 180
Lemonade fruit blends, 8 fl. oz.:
all fruit flavors *(R.W. Knudsen/Santa Cruz)* 120
all fruit flavors *(Veryfine* Chillers) 120
cherry *(Snapple)* 130
cherry, peach, or pink *(Snapple)* 120
ginger *(R.W. Knudsen* Echinacea) 100
peach or strawberry *(Snapple)* 120
tropical *(Minute Maid)* 120
Lemonade mix*, 8 fl. oz.:
(Country Time) 70
(Country Time/Kool-Aid Sugar Free) 5
(Kool-Aid Presweetened) 70
Lentil, dry, green or red *(Arrowhead Mills),* ¼ cup 150
Lentil, canned *(Eden* Organic), ½ cup 90
Lentil dishes, mix:
burgoo, spicy *(Buckeye Beans),* 1 cup* 200
cassoulet, sausage *(Buckeye Beans),* 1 cup* 170
hearty, and wild rice *(Spice Islands* Quick Meal), 1 pkg. . 190
and herb *(Eastern Traditions),* 2 oz. 160
honey baked *(Buckeye Beans),* 1 cup* 250
pilaf *(Casbah),* 1 oz. 100
pilaf, almond *(Spice Islands* Quick Meal), 1 pkg. 190
Lentil rice loaf, frozen *(Natural Touch),* 1 slice 170
Lentil salad, garden *(Cedar's),* 2 tbsp. 30
Lettuce (see also "Salad"):
Bibb or Boston, 1 head, 5 diam. 21
cos or romaine, 1 inner leaf 2
iceberg *(Dole),* ⅙ medium head, 3.2 oz. 15
iceberg, precut *(Dole),* 3 oz. 15
leaf, shredded *(Dole),* 1½ cups, 3 oz. 15
Lima beans, ½ cup, except as noted:
fresh, boiled, drained 104

Lima beans *(cont.)*

mature *(Frieda's* Christmas) 120
canned:
(S&W Butterbeans) 70
(Van Camp) 110
baby or large *(Allens* Butterbeans) 120
baby, green, or butter beans *(Stokely)* 110
green *(Allens/East Texas Fair/Sunshine)* 120
green *(Del Monte)* 80
green, w/bacon *(Trappey's* Limas) 120
w/bacon, baby white *(Trappey's* Butterbeans) 130
w/bacon, large white *(Trappey's* Butterbeans) 110
w/sausage, large white *(Trappey's* Butterbeans) . . . 110
frozen *(Seneca),* ⅔ cup 120
frozen, baby *(Green Giant Harvest Fresh)* 80
frozen, baby, butter sauce *(Green Giant),* ⅔ cup 120
frozen, Fordhook *(Birds Eye)* 100
frozen, Fordhook *(Seneca),* ⅔ cup 90
Lime *(Dole),* 1 medium, 2.4 oz. 20
Lime drink *(After the Fall* Key West), 8 fl. oz. 100
Lime juice:
fresh, 1 tbsp. 4
sweetened *(Rose's),* 1 tsp. 10
Ling, meat only, baked or broiled, 4 oz. 126
Lingcod, meat only, baked or broiled, 4 oz. 124
Linguine, refrigerated:
(Contadina), 1¼ cups 250
plain or herb *(Di Giorno),* 2.5 oz. 190
Linguine entree, frozen, and Italian sausage *(Marie
Callender),* 15 oz. 710
Liquor[1], 1 fl. oz.:
80 proof 65
90 proof 74
Liver:
beef, panfried, 4 oz. 246
chicken, simmered, 4 oz. 178
chicken, chopped, 1 cup 219

[1] Includes all pure distilled liquors: bourbon, brandy, gin, rum, Scotch,
rye, tequila, vodka, whiskey, etc.

lamb, panfried, 4 oz. 270
pork, braised, 4 oz. 187
turkey, simmered, 4 oz. 192
turkey, simmered, chopped, 1 cup 237
veal (calves'), braised, 4 oz. 187
Liver cheese *(Oscar Mayer)*, 1.3-oz. slice 120
Liver pâté, see "Pâté"
Liverwurst (see also "Braunschweiger"), 2 oz.:
(Underwood) 160
spread *(Hormel)* 130
spread *(Underwood)* 170
Lobster, northern, meat only:
boiled or steamed, 4 oz. 111
boiled or steamed, 1 cup, 5.1 oz. 142
Lobster, frozen, chunks *(Tyson* Delight), 3 oz. 80
"Lobster," imitation, frozen or refrigerated:
chunks *(Captain Jac Lobster Tasties)*, ½ cup, 3 oz. 90
salad style *(Louis Kemp Lobster Delights)*, ½ cup,
    3 oz. 80
Lobster sauce, canned *(Progresso)*, ½ cup 100
Loganberry:
fresh, 1 cup 89
canned, in light syrup *(Oregon)*, ½ cup 105
Longan, shelled, fresh, seeded, 1 oz. 17
Loquat *(Frieda's)*, 5 oz. 70
Lotus root *(Frieda's)*, 1 cup, 3 oz. 50
Lox, see "Salmon, smoked"
Lunch meat, see specific listings
Lunch meat, canned *(Spam/Spam* Less Salt), 2 oz. . . . 170
Lupin beans, in jars *(Canto* Lupini), ¼ cup 30
Lychee, shelled:
raw, peeled *(Frieda's)*, 1 oz. 18
canned, in syrup *(Ka•Me)*, 5 oz. 130
dried, 1 oz. 79
Lychee fruit juice *(Ceres* Litchi), 8 fl. oz. 120

M

FOOD AND MEASURE   **CALORIES**

Macadamia nut, shelled *(Frieda's)*, 5 pieces, 1.1 oz. 210
Macaroni (see also "Pasta")
uncooked *(Creamette)*, 2 oz. 210
uncooked, elbow, 1 cup 389
cooked, elbow, 1 cup 197
cooked, small shells, 1 cup 162
cooked, spirals, 1 cup 189
Macaroni entree, canned:
and beef *(Libby's Diner)*, 7¾ oz. 220
and cheese *(Chef Boyardee Bowl)*, 7.5 oz. 160
and cheese *(Hormel* Micro Cup)*, 7.5 oz. 260
and cheese *(Libby's Diner)*, 7¾ oz. 320
Macaroni entree, frozen:
and beef *(Freezer Queen* Homestyle), 9 oz. 220
and beef *(Lean Cuisine)*, 10 oz. 280
and beef *(Stouffer's)*, 11.5 oz. 420
and beef, w/tomato sauce *(Swanson* Lunch and More
   Casserole), 1 pkg. 270
broccoli *(Swanson Mac & More)*, 1 pkg. 220
and cheddar, white *(Swanson Mac & More)*, 1 pkg. . . . 200
and cheese *(Amy's)*, 9 oz. 450
and cheese *(Banquet)*, 9.5 oz. 320
and cheese *(Banquet* Family), 1 cup, 7 oz. 210
and cheese *(Healthy Choice)*, 9 oz. 320
and cheese *(Lean Cuisine)*, 10 oz. 290
and cheese *(Marie Callender)*, 13.5 oz. 510
and cheese *(Stouffer's* 20 oz.), approx. 1 cup, 8 oz. . . . 340
and cheese *(Swanson Mac & More* Classic), 1 pkg. . . . 240
and cheese, three, bake *(Swanson* Lunch and More
   Casserole), 1 pkg. 400
and cheese pie *(Banquet)*, 6.5 oz. 200
and cheese pie *(Morton)*, 6.5 oz. 210
w/soy cheeze *(Amy's)*, 9 oz. 360

Macaroni entree mix, and cheese:
(Creamette), 1/3 pkg. 250
(Land O Lakes Original), 1 cup* 400
(Land O Lakes Deluxe Plus), 1 cup* 360
cheddar *(Golden Grain)*, 1 cup* 340
three cheese *(Knorr* Cup), 1 pkg. 240
Mace *(McCormick)*, 1/4 tsp. 2
Mackerel, meat only, 4 oz.:
Atlantic, baked or broiled 297
king, baked or broiled 152
Pacific and jack, baked or broiled 228
Spanish, baked or broiled 179
Mackerel, canned, skinless *(Reese)*, 4.375-oz. can 240
Mackerel, smoked *(Spence & Co.)*, 2 oz. 180
Mahimahi:
fresh, see "Dolphinfish"
frozen, fillet *(Peter Pan)*, 4 oz. 100
Malanga *(Frieda's)*, 2/3 cup, 3 oz. 90
Mandarin orange, see "Tangerine"
Mango, fresh:
(Frieda's), 5 oz. 90
peeled, sliced *(Dole)*, 1/2 cup 54
Mango, dried *(Frieda's)*, 4 pieces, 1.4 oz. 130
Mango drink, cocktail *(Snapple* Madness), 8 fl. oz. 110
Mango juice *(After the Fall* Montage), 8 fl. oz. 110
Mango nectar *(Libby's/Kern's)*, 8 fl. oz. 150
Manicotti, frozen, 2 pieces:
(Celentano), 7 oz. 410
mini *(Celentano)*, 4.8 oz. 110
Manicotti entree, frozen:
cheese *(Celentano)*, 1/2 of 14-oz. pkg. 310
cheese *(Stouffer's)*, 9 oz. 380
cheese *(Weight Watchers)*, 9 1/4 oz. 260
cheese, three *(Healthy Choice)*, 11 oz. 300
Florentine *(Celentano)*, 10 oz. 220
Florentine *(Celentano* Great Choice), 10 oz. 210
Maple syrup, pure *(Cary's/MacDonald's)*, 1/4 cup 210
Margarine, 1 tbsp.:
(I Can't Believe It's Not Butter Salted/Sweet) 90
(I Can't Believe It's Not Butter Light) 50

(Land O Lakes Stick/Soft) 100
(Mazola/Mazola Unsalted) 100
(Mazola Light) 50
(Smart Beat Nonfat) 10
(Smart Beat Super Light/Trans Fat Free) 20
(Smart Beat Unsalted) 25
soft *(Parkay* Tub) 100
soft *(Parkay* Diet Tub) 50
spread *(Mazola* Light) 50
spread *(Parkay* Stick 53%) 70
spread *(Parkay* Tub 50%) 60
spread w/sweet cream, soft *(Land O Lakes* Salted) 80
spread w/sweet cream, stick *(Land O Lakes* Unsalted) . . 90
squeeze *(Parkay)* 80
whipped *(Parkay* Tub) 70
Marinade (see also "Stir-fry sauce" and specific
  listings):
(House of Tsang Classic), ½ tbsp. 15
(House of Tsang Mandarin), 1 tbsp. 25
Hawaiian *(Lawry's)*, 1 tbsp. 20
lemon butter dill *(Ken's Steak House)*, 1 tbsp. 50
lemon pepper *(Lawry's)*, 1 tbsp. 10
red wine *(Lawry's)*, 1 tbsp. 5
Marjoram *(McCormick)*, ¼ tsp. 1
Marmalade, see "Jam and preserves"
Marrow beans, dried *(Frieda's)*, ½ cup 120
Marrow squash, raw, trimmed, 1 oz. 4
Marshmallow topping, 2 tbsp.:
(Smucker's) 120
all varieties *(Marshmallow Fluff)* 60
creme *(Kraft)* 40
Mayonnaise, 1 tbsp.:
(Best Foods Real) 100
(Hellmann's/Best Foods Low Fat) 25
(Hellmann's/Best Foods Real) 100
(Kraft Real) 100
(Smart Beat Super Light Reduced Fat) 35
dressing *(Miracle Whip* Salad) 70
dressing *(Miracle Whip* Free) 15
dressing *(Miracle Whip* Light) 40

Mayonnaise *(cont.)*

dressing *(Spin Blend)*	60
dressing *(Spin Blend* Nonfat)	15
dressing *(Weight Watchers* Fat Free)	10

McDonald's, 1 serving:

breakfast items:

biscuit, plain	290
biscuit, bacon, egg, and cheese	470
biscuit, sausage	470
biscuit, sausage and egg	550
burrito	320
cinnamon roll	400
Danish, apple	360
Danish, cheese	410
Egg McMuffin	290
eggs, scrambled, 2	160
hash browns	130
hotcakes, plain	310
hotcakes, w/syrup and margarine	570
muffin, apple bran	300
muffin, English	140
sausage	170
Sausage McMuffin	360
Sausage McMuffin w/egg	440

sandwiches:

Arch Deluxe	550
Arch Deluxe w/bacon	590
Big Mac	560
cheeseburger	320
Crispy Chicken Deluxe	500
Fish Filet Deluxe	560
Grilled Chicken Deluxe	440
Grilled Chicken Deluxe, plain, w/out mayo	300
hamburger	260
Quarter Pounder	420
Quarter Pounder w/cheese	530

Chicken McNuggets:

4 pieces	190
6 pieces	290
9 pieces	430

McNuggets sauce pkt.:

   barbeque or honey 45
   honey mustard 50
   hot mustard 60
   light mayonnaise 40
   sweet and sour 50

french fries:

   small 210
   large 450
   Super Size 540

salad, garden 35
salad, grilled chicken deluxe 120
salad croutons, 1 pkg. 50

salad dressing, 1 pkg.:

   Caesar 160
   ranch 230
   red French, reduced calorie 160
   vinaigrette, lite 50

desserts and shakes:

   baked apple pie 260
   chocolate chip cookie 170
   ice cream cone, vanilla, reduced fat 150
   McDonaldland Cookies, 1 pkg. 180
   shake, chocolate, strawberry, or vanilla, small 360
   sundae, hot caramel 360
   sundae, hot fudge 340
   sundae, strawberry 290
   sundae nuts, 1/4 oz. 40

Meat, see specific listings

Meat loaf dinner, frozen:

(Banquet Extra Helping), 16 oz. 610
(Healthy Choice), 12 oz. 320
(Swanson), 1 pkg. 380
(Swanson Hungry-Man), 1 pkg. 640
tomato sauce w/ *(Morton),* 9 oz. 250

Meat loaf entree, frozen:

(Banquet), 9.5 oz. 280
and gravy, w/mashed potato *(Marie Callender),* 14 oz. . 540
and tomato sauce, vegetables *(Swanson* Lunch and
   More), 1 pkg. 270

Meat loaf entree *(cont.)*
w/whipped potato *(Lean Cuisine)*, 9⅜ oz. 240
w/whipped potato *(Stouffer's* Homestyle), 9⅞ oz. 330
"Meat" loaf mix, vegetarian *(Natural Touch)*, ¼ cup . . . 100
Meat loaf seasoning mix:
(Durkee Pouch), ⅑ pkt. 20
(Durkee/French's Roasting Bag), ⅛ pkg. 15
(Lawry's), 1 tbsp. 35
Meat spread *(Oscar Mayer* Sandwich Spread), 2 oz. . . . 130
Meat tenderizer, unseasoned *(Tone's)*, 1 tsp. 7
"Meatball," vegetarian, w/gravy, canned *(Loma Linda
     Tender Rounds)*, 6 pieces 120
Meatball entree, canned, stew:
(Dinty Moore), 1 cup 270
(Dinty Moore Cup), 7.5 oz. 250
Meatball entree, frozen (see also "Spaghetti entree"),
     Swedish:
(Healthy Choice), 9.1 oz. 280
(Marie Callender), 12.5 oz. 520
(Stouffer's), 10¼ oz. 480
(Weight Watchers), 9 oz. 300
w/pasta *(Lean Cuisine)*, 9⅛ oz. 280
Meatball sandwich, frozen, Italian *(Healthy Choice
     Hearty Handfuls)*, 6.1 oz. 320
Meatball seasoning, Italian *(Durkee* Pouch), ⅕ pkt. 20
Melon balls, frozen *(Stilwell)*, 1 cup 50
Melonberry cocktail *(Snapple)*, 8 fl. oz. 120
Menudo, canned *(Goya)*, 1 cup 200
Mesquite sauce *(S&W)*, 1 tbsp. 10
Mexican beans (see also "Chili beans"), canned,
     ½ cup:
(Chi-Chi's Ranchero) 100
(Old El Paso Mexe Beans) 110
(Stokely Red) 110
(Van Camp) 110
w/bacon and jalapeños *(Rosarita* Fiesta/3-Bean) 120
w/chicken and chilies *(Rosarita* Fiesta/3-Bean) 115
w/chilies and chorizo *(Rosarita* Fiesta/3-Bean) 110
w/jalapeños *(Allens/Brown Beauty)* 120
w/jalapeños *(Trappey's* MexiBeans) 130

w/onions and peppers *(Rosarita* Fiesta/3-Bean) 105
Mexican dinner, frozen (see also specific listings):
(Patio), 13¼ oz. 470
(Patio Fiesta), 12 oz. 350
(Patio Ranchera), 13 oz. 470
style *(Swanson Hungry-Man),* 1 pkg. 690
style, combination *(Swanson),* 1 pkg. 470
Mexican seasoning *(Chi-Chi's* Mix), 1 tsp. 10
Milk, 1 cup:
buttermilk, cultured 99
whole, 3.3% fat 150
low-fat, 2% 121
low-fat, 2%, protein fortified 137
low-fat, 1% 102
low-fat, 1%, protein fortified 119
skim, nonfat 86
Milk, canned, 2 tbsp.:
condensed, sweetened *(Carnation)* 130
condensed, sweetened, low-fat *(Eagle)* 120
condensed, sweetened, skim *(Eagle* Fat Free) 110
evaporated *(Carnation)* 40
evaporated *(Pet)* 40
evaporated, low-fat or skim *(Carnation)* 25
evaporated, skim *(Pet)* 20
Milk, chocolate, see "Chocolate milk"
"Milk," nondairy (see also "Soy beverage"), 8 fl. oz.:
(EdenBlend) 120
(Rice Dream Original/Original Enriched) 120
carob *(Rice Dream)* 150
chocolate *(Rice Dream/Rice Dream* Enriched) 170
vanilla *(Rice Dream/Rice Dream* Enriched) 130
Milkfish, meat only, baked or broiled, 4 oz. 215
Millet, cooked, 4 oz. 135
Millet flour *(Arrowhead Mills),* ¼ cup 110
Mint sauce *(Crosse & Blackwell),* 1 tsp. 5
Miso, soy, 1 tbsp.:
(Eden Hacho) 35
w/barley or brown rice *(Eden* Organic Mugi/Genmai) . . . 25
w/white rice *(Eden* Shiro) 35
Mocha drink *(Nestlé Mocha Cooler),* 1 cup 170

Molasses, 1 tbsp.:

(Grandma's 4-Star/Gold/Green) 50

blackstrap *(New Morning)* 60

Monkfish, meat only, baked or broiled, 4 oz. 110

Mortadella:

(Boar's Head Cinghiale), 2 oz. 160

w/pistachios *(Boar's Head Cinghiale),* 2 oz. 170

Muffin, 1 piece, except as noted:

(Arnold Extra Crisp) 120

apple *(Awrey's),* 1.5 oz. 130

apple *(Awrey's),* 2.5 oz. 250

banana nut *(Awrey's Grande)* 400

banana nut *(Tastykake* Family) 220

banana nut, mini *(Awrey's),* 2 pieces 200

blueberry *(Awrey's),* 1.5 oz. 130

blueberry *(Awrey's),* 2.5 oz. 210

blueberry *(Tastykake* Family) 170

blueberry, mini *(Awrey's),* 2 pieces 180

carrot raisin *(Awrey's Grande)* 360

cheese streusel *(Awrey's Grande)* 380

chocolate chocolate chip *(Awrey's Grande)* 460

corn *(Awrey's),* 1.5 oz. 130

corn *(Awrey's),* 2.5 oz. 220

corn *(Tastykake* Golden Family) 190

cranberry nut *(Awrey's)* 120

English *(Thomas')* 120

English *(Wonder)* 120

English, blueberry, cranberry, or raisin *(Thomas')* 140

English, honey wheat *(Thomas')* 110

English, oat bran or sourdough *(Thomas')* 120

English, sandwich size *(Thomas'* 4 Pack/Twin) 190

English, sourdough, sandwich size *(Thomas' Em's)* 200

lemon poppy seed *(Awrey's)* 170

lemon poppy seed, mini *(Awrey's),* 2 pieces 90

oat bran *(Hostess),* 2 pieces 320

onion, sandwich size *(Thomas' Em's)* 180

raisin *(Arnold)* 150

raisin bran *(Awrey's),* 1.5 oz. 110

raisin bran *(Awrey's),* 2.5 oz. 190

sourdough *(Arnold)* 120

Muffin mix, 1 muffin*:

all flavors *(Sweet Rewards* Fat Free) 120
apple cinnamon *(Betty Crocker* Pouch) 170
apple cinnamon *(Martha White)* 180
apple cinnamon, blueberry, or strawberry *(Pillsbury)* . . . 180
apple streusel *(Betty Crocker)* 210
banana or caramel nut *(Betty Crocker)* 170
banana nut *(Martha White)* 200
blackberry or double blueberry *(Martha White)* 180
blueberry *(Betty Crocker)* 140
blueberry *(Betty Crocker* Pouch) 160
blueberry, wild *(Betty Crocker)* 170
bran *(Martha White)* 190
bran, oat *(Martha White)* 200
chocolate chip *(Betty Crocker)* 170
chocolate chip *(Pillsbury)* 190
cinnamon streusel *(Betty Crocker)* 170
cinnamon swirl *(Duncan Hines)* 200
corn *(Betty Crocker)* 160
corn *(Gladiola)* 200
corn *(Martha White)* 180
honey pecan *(Martha White)* 180
lemon poppy seed *(Betty Crocker* Box) 190
lemon poppy seed *(Betty Crocker* Pouch) 180
lemon poppy seed *(Martha White)* 240
oatmeal raisin *(Martha White)* 200
raspberry or strawberry *(Martha White)* 180
Muffin sandwich, breakfast, frozen, eggs, bacon, and
    cheese *(Great Starts),* 1 pkg. 290
Mulberry, ½ cup 31
Mullet, striped, meat only, baked or broiled, 4 oz. 170
Mung beans, boiled, ½ cup 107
Mung beans, sprouted, raw *(Jonathan's),* 1 cup 30
Mungo beans, boiled, ½ cup 95
Mushroom, fresh:
(Dole), 5 medium, 3 oz. 20
boiled, drained, pieces, ½ cup 21
enoki, trimmed, 1 oz. 10
enoki, 1 large, 4⅛ long 2
oyster or shiitake *(Frieda's),* 3 oz. 20

Mushroom, fresh *(cont.)*
portobello *(Frieda's)*, 1 oz. 8
shiitake, cooked, 4 medium or ½ cup pieces 40
wood ear *(Frieda's)*, 3 oz. 20
yamabiko honshemeji *(Frieda's)*, ¼ cup, 1.1 oz. 10
Mushroom, canned, ½ cup, except as noted:
(Seneca/Seneca No Salt/Shiitake) 25
(Seneca Jars) 30
all varieties *(Green Giant)* 30
all varieties, except with garlic *(BinB)*, 1 can 30
with garlic *(BinB)*, 1 can 35
teriyaki, sliced *(Seneca)* 80
Mushroom, dried:
chanterelle *(Frieda's)*, 2 pieces 15
morel *(Frieda's)*, 3 pieces 15
porcini *(Frieda's)*, 5 pieces 15
shiitake, 4 medium, .5 oz. 44
stir-fry *(Frieda's)*, 4 pieces 15
straw, padi *(Frieda's)*, 6 pieces 15
Mushroom, frozen, shiitake *(Seneca)*, ½ cup 20
Mushroom, marinated *(Seneca)*, 1 oz. 90
Mushroom, pickled *(Seneca)*, 1 oz. 5
Mushroom blends:
pasta or soup *(Frieda's)*, 6 pieces 15
poultry, sauce, or steak *(Frieda's)*, 4 pieces 15
Mushroom gravy, ¼ cup:
canned *(Heinz Homestyle* Fat Free) 10
canned, country or w/wine *(Pepperidge Farm)* 30
canned, regular or creamy *(Franco-American)* 20
mix* *(Durkee)* 15
mix* *(French's)* 10
Mushroom salad *(Seneca)*, 1 tbsp. 5
Mushroom sauce *(House of Tsang)*, 1 tbsp. 10
Mussel, blue, meat only, boiled or steamed, 4 oz. 195
Mustard, prepared, 1 tsp., except as noted:
(Boar's Head Deli) 0
(French's Yellow) 0
(Grey Poupon Dijon/Deli/Spicy) 5
(Gulden's Spicy) 0
(Hunt's) 3

all varieties *(Nance's)* 15
Chinese *(House of Tsang)*, 1 pkt. 15
Dijon *(Roland* Extra Strong) 10
Dijon, honey *(Grey Poupon)* 10
Mustard blend *(Best Foods/Hellmann's Dijonnaise)*,
   1 tsp. 5
Mustard cabbage *(Frieda's* Gai Choy), 1 cup, 3 oz. 20
Mustard greens:
fresh, chopped, boiled, drained, ½ cup 11
canned *(Allens/Sunshine)*, ½ cup 30
Mustard sauce mix, herb *(Knorr)*, 1 tbsp. 4
Mustard seed, yellow *(McCormick)*, ¼tsp. 2
Mustard spinach, boiled, drained, chopped, ½ cup 14

N

FOOD AND MEASURE   **CALORIES**

Nacho dip mix (see also "Cheese dip") *(Knorr),* ½ tsp. . . . 10
Natto, ½ cup 187
Navy beans, ½ cup:
dry, boiled 129
canned *(Eden* Organic) 110
canned *(Stokely)* 110
canned, w/bacon or w/bacon/jalapeños *(Trappey's)* . . . 110
Navy beans, sprouted, raw, ½ cup 35
Nectarine, fresh:
(Dole), 1 fruit, 5 oz. 70
sliced, ½ cup 34
New England sausage *(Oscar Mayer),* 1.6 oz. 60
Newburg sauce mix *(Knorr),* ⅓ pkg. 30
Noodle, Chinese:
(Nasoya), 1 cup, 2¾ oz. 210
cellophane or long rice, dry, 2 oz. 199
chow mein *(Frieda's),* 4 oz. 270
chow mein *(La Choy/Chun King),* ¼ cup 140
crispy, wide *(La Choy),* ½ cup 150
egg, dried *(House of Tsang),* 2 oz. 200
rice *(La Choy),* ½ cup 120
Noodle, egg:
uncooked, all varieties *(Creamette/Goodman's),* 2 oz. . . . 220
uncooked, bow ties *(Mueller's),* 2 oz. 220
cooked, 1 cup 212
Noodle, egg-free, frozen *(Morningstar Farms*
    Homestyle),* ½ cup 160
Noodle, Japanese, dry, except as noted:
soba *(Eden* Organic Traditional),* ½ cup 200
soba, buckwheat *(Eden* 40%),* 2 oz. 190
soba, cooked, 1 cup 113
lotus root, mugwort, traditional, or wild yam *(Eden),*
    2 oz. 190

Noodle, Japanese *(cont.)*
plain or spinach *(Nasoya)*, 1 cup, 2¾ oz. 210
somen *(Eden* Organic Traditional), ½ cup 200
somen, cooked, 1 cup 230
udon *(Eden* Organic Traditional), ½ cup 200
udon, cooked, 4 oz. 115
Noodle dishes, canned or frozen, see "Noodle entree"
Noodle dishes, mix, 1 cup*:
Alfredo *(Lipton* Noodles & Sauce) 330
Alfredo, broccoli *(Lipton* Noodles & Sauce) 340
beef *(Lipton* Noodles & Sauce) 280
butter *(Lipton* Noodles & Sauce) 310
butter and herb *(Lipton* Noodles & Sauce) 300
chicken *(Lipton* Noodles & Sauce) 290
chicken, broccoli *(Lipton* Noodles & Sauce) 310
chicken, creamy *(Lipton* Noodles & Sauce) 320
chicken tetrazzini *(Lipton* Noodles & Sauce) 300
Oriental *(Pasta Roni)* 290
Parmesan *(Lipton* Noodles & Sauce) 330
sour cream and chives *(Lipton* Noodles & Sauce) 310
Stroganoff *(Lipton* Noodles & Sauce) 300
Noodle entree, canned, 1 cup, except as noted:
w/beef *(Hunt's* Homestyle) 150
w/beef *(La Choy* Bi-Pack) 155
w/chicken *(Hormel* Micro Cup), 7½ oz. 200
w/chicken *(Hormel* Micro Cup), 10½ oz. 270
w/chicken *(Hunt's* Homestyle) 175
w/chicken *(La Choy* Bi-Pack) 155
sweet and sour, w/chicken *(La Choy* Entree) 260
w/vegetables *(La Choy* Entree) 130
w/vegetables and beef *(La Choy* Entree) 160
w/vegetables and chicken *(La Choy* Entree) 160
Noodle entree, frozen:
escalloped, and chicken *(Marie Callender)*, 1 cup,
   6.5 oz. 420
Romanoff *(Stouffer's)*, 12 oz. 490
Nut topping (see also specific listings) *(Planters)*,
   2 tbsp. 100
Nutmeg, ground *(McCormick)*, ¼ tsp. 3
Nuts, see specific listings

Nuts, mixed, 1 oz.:
dry- or oil-roasted *(Planters/Planters* Deluxe) 170
honey-roasted *(Planters)* 140
oil-roasted, w/peanuts 175
sesame, oil-roasted *(Planters)* 150
tamari-roasted *(Eden)* 170

O

Oat (see also "Cereal"):
flakes, rolled *(Arrowhead Mills)*, ⅓ cup 130
rolled or oatmeal, cooked, 1 cup 145
steel cut *(Arrowhead Mills)*, ¼ cup 170
Oat bran, dry *(Arrowhead Mills)*, ⅓ cup 150
Ocean perch, Atlantic, meat only, baked or broiled,
    4 oz. 137
Octopus, meat only, boiled or steamed, 4 oz. 186
Octopus, canned:
(Goya), ¼ cup 140
in olive oil *(Goya)*, ¼ cup 150
Oil, 1 tbsp., except as noted:
butter oil 112
canola, corn, hazelnut, olive, palm, peanut, safflower,
    sesame, soybean, sunflower, vegetable, or walnut . . . 120
cod liver or herring 123
Oriental cooking or sesame *(House of Tsang)*, 1 tsp. 45
salmon or sardine 123
Oil substitute *(Baking Healthy)*, 1 tbsp. 30
Okra:
fresh, boiled, drained, 8 pods, 3 ∞⅝ 27
canned, Creole gumbo *(Trappey's)*, ½ cup 35
canned, cut or w/tomatoes *(Allens/Trappey's)*, ½ cup 25
canned, w/tomatoes and corn *(Allens/Trappey's)*, ½ cup . . 30
frozen, whole *(Stilwell)*, 9 pods, 3 oz. 35
frozen, and tomatoes *(Stilwell)*, ⅔ cup 25
Old-fashioned loaf *(Oscar Mayer)*, 1 oz. 70
Olive, pickled:
black, see "ripe," below
Calamata *(Krinos)*, 3 pieces 45
green, w/pits, 10 large 45
green, cracked *(Krinos)*, ½ oz. 20
green, queen/Spanish *(S&W)*, 2 pieces 20

Olive *(cont.)*
green, salad *(B&G)*, 2 tbsp. 25
ripe, w/pits *(S&W)*, 1 super colossal 15
ripe, pitted *(Musco Black Pearls)*, 5 pieces, ½ oz. 25
ripe, pitted *(S&W)*, 3 extra large or jumbo 25
ripe, pitted *(Vlasic)*, 4 large or 6 small 25
ripe, pitted, Spanish *(Vlasic)*, 8 small 20
ripe, oil-cured *(Progresso)*, 3 pieces 70
royal *(Krinos)*, ½ oz. 30
stuffed, Manzanilla *(S&W)*, 3 pieces 25
stuffed, queen *(Vlasic)*, ½ oz. 20
stuffed, w/tuna *(Goya)*, 4 pieces 25
Olive loaf *(Boar's Head)*, 2 oz. 130
Olive oil, see "Oil"
Olive salad, in jars:
(Goya), ¼ cup 25
drained *(Progresso)*, 2 tbsp. 25
Onion, mature:
fresh, raw, chopped, ½ cup 30
fresh, raw, cipolline *(Frieda's)*, 3 pieces, 3 oz. 35
fresh, raw, pearl *(Frieda's)*, ⅔ cup, 3 oz. 30
fresh, raw, Vidalia, chopped *(Dole)*, ½ cup 30
fresh, boiled, drained, chopped, ½ cup 47
canned, whole *(Green Giant)*, ½ cup 35
canned, whole *(S&W)*, ½ cup 40
canned, cocktail *(S&W 4 oz.)*, 12 pieces, 1.1 oz. 5
canned, Vidalia, sweet, in sauce *(Boar's Head)*, 1 tbsp. . . 10
frozen *(Seneca)*, ⅔ cup 30
frozen, chopped *(Ore-Ida)*, ¾ cup 25
frozen, rings, see "Onion rings"
Onion, dried, flakes, 1 tbsp. 16
Onion, green (scallion), raw, trimmed, w/top:
chopped, ½ cup 16
chopped *(Dole)*, ¼ cup, .9 oz. 10
Onion dip, 2 tbsp.:
creamy *(Kraft* Premium) 45
French *(Frito-Lay)* 60
French *(Heluva* Good) 50
French *(Heluva* Good Free) 25
French *(Old Dutch)* 50

French *(Ruffle's)* 70
French *(Ruffle's* Low Fat) 40
French *(Sealtest)* 50
sour cream and *(Lay's* Low Fat) 40
Onion dip mix, and chive *(Knorr)*, ½tsp. 5
Onion gravy, ¼ cup:
canned, zesty *(Heinz* Homestyle) 25
mix* *(Durkee)* 10
mix* *(French's)* 15
mix*, brown, Lyonnaise *(Knorr)* 20
Onion powder *(McCormick)*, ¼ tsp. 3
Onion rings:
canned *(French's French Fried Real Onions)*, 2 tbsp. 45
frozen *(Mrs. Paul's* Old Fashioned), 7 rings, 3 oz. 230
frozen *(Ore-Ida Onion Ringers)*, 6 rings 230
Onion sprouts *(Jonathan's)*, 1 cup 30
Opo squash *(Frieda's)*, ⅔ cup, 3 oz. 10
Orange, fresh:
(Dole), 1 medium 50
blood *(Frieda's)*, 5 oz. 70
California navel, 2⅞ -diam. orange 65
California Valencia, 2⅝ -diam. orange 59
Florida, 2¹¹⁄₁₆ -diam. orange 69
Orange, mandarin, see "Tangerine"
Orange drink, 8 fl. oz.:
(Snapple Orangeade) 120
chilled or frozen* *(Bright & Early)* 120
mix* *(Tang)* 100
Orange drink blends, 8 fl. oz.:
all varieties *(Dole)* 120
all varieties, except cranberry, peach-strawberry, and
    strawberry-banana *(Tropicana Twister)* 120
cranberry, peach-strawberry, and strawberry-banana
    (Tropicana Twister) 130
guava nectar *(Kern's)* 150
pineapple *(Lincoln)* 130
tropic *(Snapple)* 120
Orange juice, 8 fl. oz., except as noted:
fresh, 6 fl. oz. 83
(Apple & Eve), 10 fl. oz. 130

Orange juice *(cont.)*
(R.W. Knudsen) 100
(S&W), 6-fl.-oz. can 90
(Seneca) 120
(Snapple Grove), 12 fl. oz. 170
(Tropicana Pure Premium/*Season's Best)* 110
(Veryfine) 120
all varieties, except calcium rich *(Minute Maid*
  Premium) 110
calcium rich *(Minute Maid* Premium) 120
Orange juice blends, 8 fl. oz.:
kiwi–passion fruit *(Tropicana* Tropics) 100
peach-mango *(Tropicana* Tropics) 110
pineapple or strawberry banana *(Tropicana* Tropics) 110
punch *(Veryfine* Juice-Ups) 140
Orange peel, candied *(S&W)*, 58 pieces, 1.1 oz. 80
Orange peel salsa, all varieties *(Sorrell Ridge)*, 2 tbsp. . . 12
Orange sauce, mandarin *(Ka•Me)*, 2 tbsp. 80
Oregano, dried, 1 tsp. 3
Oriental 5-spice *(Tone's)*, 1 tsp. 9
Oriental sauce (see also specific listings):
(House of Tsang Chow Chow), 1 tsp. 5
(House of Tsang Imperial), 1 tbsp. 25
(House of Tsang Namasu), 1 tsp. 10
brown, spicy *(House of Tsang)*, 1 tsp. 15
hot and spicy *(House of Tsang* Hunan), 1 tsp. 5
Oyster, fresh, meat only:
Eastern, wild, raw, 6 medium, 3 oz. 57
Eastern, wild, baked or broiled, 4 oz. 82
Eastern, wild, steamed or poached, 4 oz. 155
Eastern, farmed, baked or broiled, 4 oz. 90
Pacific, raw, boiled, or steamed, 1 medium 41
Pacific, boiled or steamed, 4 oz. 185
Oyster, canned:
whole *(S&W)*, 2 oz. 70
smoked *(S&W)*, 2 oz. 100
Oyster plant, see "Salsify"
Oyster-shrimp sauce *(TryMe* Caribbean Clipper), 1 tsp. . . 10
Oyster stew, see "Soup"

P–Q

FOOD AND MEASURE   **CALORIES**

Palm, hearts of *(Haddon House)*, 4.5 oz. 20
Pancake, frozen, 3 pieces, except as noted:
(Aunt Jemima Original) 200
(Downyflake) 270
(Hungry Jack Microwave Original) 270
blueberry *(Aunt Jemima)* 210
blueberry *(Hungry Jack* Microwave) 230
buttermilk *(Aunt Jemima)* 180
buttermilk *(Hungry Jack* Microwave) 280
buttermilk, mini *(Hungry Jack* Microwave), 11 pieces . . 260
silver dollar *(Great Starts)*, 7 pieces 290
Pancake breakfast, frozen, 1 pkg.:
w/bacon *(Great Starts)* 400
w/sausage *(Great Starts)* 490
silver dollar, w/sausage *(Great Starts)* 340
Pancake mix, 1/3 cup mix, except as noted:
(Aunt Jemima Original) 150
(Aunt Jemima Complete/Buttermilk Complete) 190
(Betty Crocker Complete/Buttermilk Complete) 200
(Bisquick Shake 'N Pour Original/Blueberry), 1/2 cup . . . 210
(Gladiola), 1/2 cup 240
(Hungry Jack Original) 150
(Hungry Jack Premeasured), 1/2 pkt. 200
(Hungry Jack Extra Lights) 160
(Hungry Jack Extra Lights Complete) 150
(Martha White Flapstax), 1/2 cup 240
buckwheat *(Arrowhead Mills)* 140
buttermilk *(Hungry Jack/Hungry Jack* Complete) 160
buttermilk *(Robin Hood)* 180
whole wheat *(Aunt Jemima)*, 1/4 cup 130
Pancake syrup (see also "Maple syrup"), 1/4 cup:
(Log Cabin) 200
(Log Cabin Lite) 100

Pancake syrup *(cont.)*
all flavors *(Hungry Jack)* 210
all flavors *(Hungry Jack* Lite) 100
all flavors *(S&W* Reduced Calorie) 60
Pancreas, braised:
beef, 4 oz. 307
veal (calf), 4 oz. 290
Papaya:
fresh, 1-lb. papaya, 3½ ∞5⅛ 117
fresh, peeled and cubed *(Dole),* ½ cup 27
canned, in light syrup *(Ka•Me),* ¾ cup 120
frozen, slices *(Goya),* ⅓ pkg. 50
Papaya, dried *(Frieda's),* ⅓ cup, 1.4 oz. 140
Papaya drink, 8 fl. oz., except as noted:
(Farmer's Market) 130
colada *(Snapple)* 120
nectar *(Libby's/Kern's),* 11.5 fl. oz. 210
nectar *(Santa Cruz)* 110
Pappadum *(Patak's),* 3 pieces 80
Paprika, 1 tsp. 6
Parsley:
fresh, 10 sprigs 4
fresh, chopped, ½ cup 11
dried *(McCormick),* ¼ tsp. . . . . <1
Parsley root *(Frieda's),* ⅔ cup, 3 oz. 10
Parsnip, boiled, 1 medium, 9 ∞2¼ diam. 130
Passion fruit, fresh *(Frieda's),* 5 oz. 140
Passion fruit juice *(Snapple* Supreme), 10 fl. oz. 160
Passion fruit–mango drink *(Heinke's),* 8 fl. oz. 130
Pasta, dry, uncooked (see also "Macaroni"), 2 oz.:
all varieties *(Creamette/Prince)* 210
all varieties *(Delverde)* 200
all varieties, w/egg *(Herb's)* 220
shells *(Goya* Conchas) 210
spaghetti *(Eden* Organic) 200
spaghetti, whole wheat *(Eden* Organic) 210
spirals, spinach *(Eden* Organic) 210
tricolor *(Mueller's)* 210
vegetable *(Eden* Organic) 210

Pasta, dry, cooked:
plain, 1 cup 197
corn, 1 cup 176
spinach, 1 cup 183
whole wheat, 1 cup 174
Pasta, refrigerated, see specific listings
Pasta dinner, frozen, w/beef and broccoli *(Marie Callender),* 15 oz. 570
Pasta dishes, mix (see also specific listings), 1 cup*:
Alfredo primavera *(Land O Lakes)* 350
butter and herb *(Lipton* Pasta & Sauce) 270
cheese, cheddar, mild *(Lipton* Pasta & Sauce) 290
cheese, cheddar broccoli *(Lipton* Pasta & Sauce) 340
cheese, four, corkscrews *(Pasta Roni)* 410
cheese, four, Parmesano *(Land O Lakes)* 340
chicken, herb Parmesan *(Lipton* Pasta & Sauce) 280
chicken, roasted garlic *(Lipton* Pasta & Sauce) 290
chicken, stir-fry *(Lipton* Pasta & Sauce) 270
garlic, creamy *(Lipton* Pasta & Sauce) 350
garlic, roasted, w/tomatoes *(Lipton* Pasta & Sauce) . . . 270
herb, savory, w/garlic *(Lipton* Pasta & Sauce) 280
Italian herb butter *(Land O Lakes)* 340
mushroom, creamy *(Lipton* Pasta & Sauce) 320
sun-dried tomato basil pesto *(Land O Lakes)* 330
Pasta entree, canned, see specific pasta listings
Pasta entree, frozen (see also specific listings):
cheddar bake w/ *(Lean Cuisine),* 9 oz. 260
cheddar w/beef and tomatoes *(Stouffer's),* 11 oz. 450
w/cheddar and broccoli *(Banquet),* 9.5 oz. 330
and Italian sausage *(Banquet* Family Size), 1 cup . . . 340
primavera Alfredo *(Lean Cuisine Lunch Classics),*
    10 oz. 300
w/sausage and peppers *(Banquet),* 9.5 oz. 300
and spinach Romano *(Weight Watchers* International
    Selections), 10.4 oz. 240
stuffed trio *(Marie Callender),* 10.5 oz. 380
vegetable Italiano *(Healthy Choice),* 10 oz. 250
Pasta sauce, tomato (see also specific listings),
    ¹/₂ cup:
(Del Monte Traditional) 60

Pasta sauce *(cont.)*

(*Healthy Choice* Traditional) 50
(*Paesana* Casalinga) 70
(*Patsy's* Fileto di Pomodoro) 90
(*Prego* Low Sodium/No Salt Added) 110
(*Prego* Traditional) 140
(*Prego Extra Chunky* Tomato Supreme) 120
all varieties (*Del Monte* Chunky) 60
all varieties (*Del Monte D'Italia*) 50
w/basil (*Barilla*) 70
w/basil (*Classica* Di Napoli) 50
w/basil (*Prego/Prego Extra Chunky* Zesty) 110
cheese, four (*Classico* Di Parma) 70
cheese, three (*Prego*) 100
cheese and garlic, Italian (*Hunt's*) 65
garden combination (*Prego Extra Chunky*) 90
garlic (*Prego Extra Chunky* Supreme) 130
garlic, roasted:
   (*Healthy Choice*) 50
   and Romano (*Healthy Choice*) 60
   and sun-dried tomatoes (*Healthy Choice*) 50
garlic and cheese (*Prego Extra Chunky*) 120
garlic and herb (*Healthy Choice*) 50
garlic and mushroom (*Healthy Choice*) 45
garlic and onion (*Healthy Choice*) 40
garlic-onion or green pepper–mushroom (*Del Monte*) . . . 60
hot (*Pomodoro Fresca* Cayenne) 40
Italian spice (*Aunt Millie's* Family Style) 90
marinara (*Aunt Millie's*) 70
marinara (*Barilla*) 80
marinara (*Hunt's* Chunky) 60
marinara (*Paesana*) 115
marinara (*Prego*) 110
marinara (*Progresso*) 80
marinara (*Progresso* Authentic) 90
marinara, w/burgundy (*Healthy Choice*) 50
meat (*Aunt Millie's*) 80
meat flavor (*Progresso*) 100
meat flavored (*Prego*) 140
meat or mushroom (*Del Monte*) 70

mushroom *(Aunt Millie's)* 70
mushroom *(Healthy Choice* Super Chunky) 40
mushroom *(Prego)* 150
mushroom *(Prego Extra Chunky* Supreme) 130
mushroom *(Progresso* Chunky) 80
mushroom and diced onion or tomato *(Prego Extra*
   Chunky) 110
mushroom and garlic *(Barilla)* 80
mushroom and garlic or sweet pepper *(Healthy Choice*
   Super Chunky) 45
mushroom and green pepper *(Prego Extra Chunky)* 120
mushroom and ripe olive *(Classico* Di Sicilia) 50
mushroom w/extra spice *(Prego Extra Chunky)* 120
olive, green and black *(Barilla)* 100
w/olives and mushrooms *(Classico Di Sicilia)* 50
onion and garlic *(Classico* Di Sorrento) 80
onion and garlic *(Prego/Prego Extra Chunky)* 110
Parmesan or mushroom Parmesan *(Prego)* 120
pepper, sweet, and onion *(Classico* Di Salerno) 70
pepper, sweet, spicy *(Barilla)* 80
pepper, sweet, spicy *(Classico* Di Roma Arrabbiata) 60
w/pesto *(Classico* Di Genoa) 110
sausage, Italian, and fennel *(Classico D'Abruzzi)* 90
sausage, pepper, and mushroom *(Porino's)* 150
spinach and cheese *(Classico* Di Firenze) 80
sun-dried tomato *(Classico* Di Capri) 80
sun-dried tomato and herb *(Healthy Choice)* 60
vegetable primavera *(Healthy Choice* Super Chunky) 45
vegetables *(Prego Extra Chunky* Supreme) 90
vegetables, Italian *(Hunt's* Old Country) 65
vegetables, Italian style *(Healthy Choice)* 40
zucchini and Parmesan *(Classico* Di Milano) 70
Pasta sauce, refrigerated, tomato (see also specific
   listings):
cheese, four *(Di Giorno)*, ¼ cup 200
marinara *(Contadina)*, ½ cup 80
marinara *(Di Giorno)*, ½ cup 100
meat, traditional *(Di Giorno)*, ½ cup 120
olive oil and garlic, w/cheese *(Di Giorno)*, ¼ cup 370
primavera *(Tutta Pasta)*, ½ cup 130

Pasta sauce, refrigerated *(cont.)*
puttanesca *(Tutta Pasta)*, ½ cup 100
red bell pepper *(Contadina)*, ½ cup 180
roasted garlic–artichoke *(Monterey Pasta Company)*,
  ½ cup 70
tomato, basil or chunky *(Contadina* Fat Free)*, ½ cup . . . 45
tomato, plum, and basil *(Contadina)*, ½ cup 70
vodka *(Tutta Pasta)*, ½ cup 300
Pasta sauce mix (see also specific listings):
(Lawry's), 1 tbsp. 35
garlic and herb *(Knorr)*, ⅓ pkg. 70
salad *(Durkee* Pouch)*, 2 tsp. 10
Pastrami (see also "Turkey pastrami"), beef:
(Healthy Choice), 2 oz. 60
(Healthy Deli), 2 oz. 80
brisket or Romanian *(Boar's Head)*, 2 oz. 90
round *(Boar's Head)*, 2 oz. 70
Pastry shell, frozen (see also "Pie crust"):
patty *(Pepperidge Farm)*, 1 shell 230
sheet, puff *(Pepperidge Farm)*, ⅙ sheet 200
tart shell *(Oronoque)*, 3 shell 140
tart shell *(Pet-Ritz)*, ¼ of 6 shell 110
Pâté, liver (see also "Liverwurst"), canned:
(Sells), ¼ cup 160
chicken liver *(Chef Giovanni's)*, 2 oz. 190
chicken liver, 1 tbsp. 26
goose liver, smoked, 1 tbsp. 60
Pea pod, Chinese, see "Peas, edible-podded"
Peach:
fresh, 2½ -diam. peach, 4 per lb. 37
fresh, pulp, sliced, ½ cup 37
canned, ½ cup, except as noted:
  (Hunt's) 100
  (S&W Ready-Cut California/Tropical Sun)* 80
  w/cinnamon *(S&W Sweet Memory* Ready-Cut Sun)* . . 70
  in juice, cling *(Libby's* Lite)* 60
  in juice, cling *(S&W* Natural)* 80
  in juice or extra light syrup *(Del Monte* Lite)* . . . 60
  in heavy syrup *(Del Monte/Del Monte* Melba)* 100
  in heavy syrup *(S&W)* 100

raspberry or harvest spice flavor *(Del Monte)* 80
spiced *(S&W)*, 4.3-oz. piece 100
spiced, whole *(Del Monte)* 100
frozen, sliced *(Stilwell)*, 1 cup 60
Peach, dried *(Sonoma)*, 3–5 pieces, 1.4 oz. 120
Peach drink, 8 fl. oz.:
(After the Fall) 100
(Dole) 140
(Tree Top Quake) 120
Peach dumpling, frozen *(Pepperidge Farm)*, 1 piece . . . 300
Peach juice *(Snapple* Dixie), 12 fl. oz. 170
Peach nectar *(Libby's)*, 8 fl. oz. 150
Peach salsa *(Sorrell Ridge)*, 2 tbsp. 12
Peanut, shelled, 1 oz., except as noted:
dry-roasted *(Little Debbie)* 160
dry-roasted or honey-roasted *(Planters)* 160
honey-roasted *(Frito-Lay)*, ¼ cup 270
honey-roasted, oil-roasted *(Planters* Reduced Fat) 130
hot and spicy *(Planters Heat)* 160
oil-roasted *(Pennant)* 170
oil-roasted *(Planters/Planters* Munch 'N Go) 170
oil-roasted, fancy *(Paradise/White Swan)*, ¼ cup,
1½ oz. 270
salted *(Frito-Lay)* 370
Spanish *(Planters)* 170
sweet *(Planters Sweet N Crunchy)* 140
Peanut butter, 2 tbsp.:
(Knott's All Natural Crunchy) 190
*(Laura Scudder's/*Reduced Fat/Unsalted) 200
(Smuckers Natural/Reduced Fat) 200
all varieties *(Jif/Jif* Reduced Fat/*Simply Jif)* 190
all varieties *(Skippy)* 190
creamy or crunchy *(Peter Pan/Peter Pan Plus)* 190
creamy or crunchy *(Smart Choice)* 195
whipped, creamy or crunchy *(Peter Pan)* 140
Peanut sauce, Oriental:
(House of Tsang Bangkok Padang), 1 tbsp. 45
cooking *(Kylin Singapore Satay)*, ¼ cup 60
Pear, ½ cup, except as noted:
fresh, Bartlett, 1 medium, 2½ per lb. 98

Pear *(cont.)*

fresh, sliced 49
canned *(S&W Ready-Cut California Sun)* 80
canned, in juice *(Libby's Lite)* 60
canned, in juice or extra light syrup *(Del Monte)* 60
canned, Bartlett, in juice *(S&W Natural)* 80
canned, in heavy syrup *(Del Monte)* 100
canned, Bartlett, in heavy syrup *(S&W)* 90
canned, ginger flavor *(Del Monte)* 90
Pear, Asian *(Frieda's)*, 5 oz. 60
Pear, dried *(Sonoma)*, 3–4 pieces, 1.4 oz. 120
Pear juice, 8 fl. oz.:
(After the Fall Harvest) 90
(Heinke's Organic/*R.W. Knudsen* Organic) 120
Pear nectar *(Libby's)*, 8 fl. oz. 150
Peas, crowder, ½ cup:
canned *(Allens/East Texas Fair/Homefolks)* 110
frozen *(Stilwell)* 120
Peas, edible-podded:
fresh, boiled, drained, ½ cup 34
fresh, snow *(Frieda's)*, 1 cup, 3 oz. 35
fresh, sugar snap *(Frieda's)*, ⅔ cup, 3 oz. 35
frozen, snap *(Seneca)*, ⅔ cup 45
frozen, snow *(La Choy)*, 3 oz., about 35 pods 35
frozen, sugar snap *(Green Giant)*, ¾ cup 35
frozen, sugar snap *(Green Giant Harvest Fresh)*, ⅔ cup . . 50
Peas, field, canned, ½ cup:
fresh shell *(Allens/East Texas Fair/Homefolks)* 120
dry, w/bacon *(Trappey's)* 90
dry, w/snaps and bacon *(Trappey's)* 110
Peas, green, fresh:
(Dole), 2.5 oz. 30
raw, in the pod, 1 lb. 140
boiled, drained, ½ cup 67
Peas, green, canned, ½ cup:
(Del Monte/Del Monte No Salt) 60
(S&W Petit Pois/Sweet) 70
(Seneca/Seneca No Salt) 70
(Stokely/Stokely No Salt) 60
all varieties *(Green Giant/Green Giant LeSueur)* 60

early June, dry *(Crest Top)* 100
very young, small *(Del Monte)* 60
and carrots *(Green Giant)* 50
and carrots *(S&W)* 50
w/mushrooms and pearl onions *(LeSueur)* 60
w/pearl onions *(Green Giant)* 60
w/pearl onions *(S&W)* 40
Peas, green, dried *(Frieda's)*, ⅓ cup, 3 oz. 130
Peas, green, frozen, ⅔ cup, except as noted:
(Seabrook) 70
(Seneca) 80
baby sweet or early June *(Green Giant LeSueur)* 60
sweet *(Green Giant)* 70
sweet *(Green Giant Harvest Fresh)* 60
in butter sauce *(Green Giant LeSueur)*, ¾ cup 100
and carrots *(Seneca)* 50
and mushrooms *(Green Giant LeSueur)*, ¾ cup 60
and onions *(Seneca)* 70
and pearl onions *(Green Giant)* 60
and pearl onions *(Green Giant Harvest Fresh)*, ½ cup . . 50
potatoes, carrots *(Green Giant American Mixtures)* 70
Peas, lady, canned, w/snaps *(East Texas Fair)*, ½ cup . 100
Peas, pepper, canned *(Allens/East Texas Fair)*, ½ cup . 120
Peas, purple hull, ½ cup:
canned *(East Texas)* 120
frozen *(Stilwell)* 110
Peas, snow or sugar snap, see "Peas, edible-podded"
Peas, split, see "Split peas"
Peas, sweet, see "Peas, green"
Peas, white acre, canned *(East Texas Fair)*, ½ cup 100
Pecan, shelled:
chips *(Planters)*, 2-oz. pkg. 390
halves or pieces *(Planters)*, 1 oz. 190
honey-roasted *(Planters)*, 1 oz. 180
Pecan topping, w/syrup *(Smucker's)*, 2 tbsp. 170
Penne, refrigerated *(Tutta Pasta)*, 1 cup 290
Penne dishes, mix:
Alfredo *(Knorr)*, ¾ cup 280
w/sun-dried tomato Parmesan *(Knorr)*, ½ cup 270

Penne entree, frozen:
(Healthy Choice), 8 oz. 230
and pepperoni *(Marie Callender),* 15 oz. 800
Pepper, seasoning:
black, red, or cayenne, ground, 1 tsp. 6
black, whole, 1 tsp. 8
white *(McCormick),* ¼ tsp. 2
Pepper, banana, mild *(Nalley)* 1 oz. 5
Pepper, bell, see "Pepper, sweet"
Pepper, cherry:
(Trappey's), 2 pieces 10
hot *(Progresso),* 1-oz. piece 10
hot, sliced, drained *(Progresso),* 2 tbsp. 25
sweet *(Nalley),* 1 oz. 10
Pepper, chili, fresh:
all varieties *(Frieda's),* 1.1-oz. piece 10
raw, green and red, chopped, ½ cup 30
Pepper, chili, in jars:
chopped, w/liquid, ½ cup 17
green, whole *(Chi-Chi's),* 1 chili 10
green, whole, peeled *(Old El Paso),* 1 chili 10
green, chopped *(Old El Paso),* 2 tbsp. 5
green, diced *(Chi-Chi's),* 2 tbsp. 10
green, diced or strips *(Rosarita),* 2 tbsp. 5
yellow, hot *(Del Monte),* 4 pieces, 1 oz. 10
Pepper, chilpotle, sauce, *(Del Monte),* 2 tbsp. 20
Pepper, jalapeño:
fresh, whole *(Frieda's),* 1 piece, 1.1 oz. 10
canned or in jars:
    (Trappey's), 2 pieces 10
    whole, w/escabeche *(Rosarita),* ¼ cup 8
    diced *(Rosarita),* 2 tbsp. 5
    marinated *(La Victoria),* 1.1 oz. 10
    nacho, sliced *(Rosarita),* 1.1 oz., 2 tbsp. 5
    peeled *(Old El Paso),* 3 pieces, 1.1 oz. 5
    pickled *(Old El Paso),* 2 tbsp. 2
    sliced *(Old El Paso),* 1.1 oz., 2 tbsp. 10
    nacho, sliced *(Del Monte),* 1 oz., 2 tbsp. 5
Pepper, nacho, pickled *(Goya),* 14 slices 10
Pepper, roasted, see "Pepper, sweet, in jars"

Pepper, serrano, fresh *(Frieda's)*, 1.1-oz. piece 10
Pepper, sweet, fresh:
green *(Dole)*, 1 medium, 5.3 oz. 30
green and red, raw, chopped, ½ cup 13
green and red, boiled, drained, chopped, ½ cup 19
yellow, raw, 1 large, 5 ∞3 diam. 50
yellow, raw, 10 strips, 1.8 oz. 14
Pepper, sweet, in jars:
filet *(Hebrew National/Rosoff/Shorr's)*, 1 oz. 9
fried, drained *(Progresso)*, 2 tbsp. 60
roasted *(Progresso)*, 1 oz. 10
roasted, fire, w/garlic, oil *(Paesana)*, 2 tbsp. 20
sun-dried, marinated *(Antica Italia)*, 1 oz. 170
Pepper, sweet, frozen, red *(Seneca)*, ¾ cup 25
Pepper salad *(B&G)*, 1 oz. 10
Pepper sauce (see also specific listings), hot:
(Gebhardt), 1 tsp. 0
all varieties *(Tabasco)*, 1 tsp. 0
Pepper steak, see "Beef entree"
Pepperoncini *(Zorba)*, 5 pieces, 1.1 oz. 15
Pepperoni:
(Hormel/Leoni/Rosa Grande), 1 oz. 140
(Patrick Cudahy 3 oz.), 16 slices, 1.1 oz. 150
Perch (see also "Ocean perch"), meat only, baked or
broiled, 4 oz. 133
Persimmon, fresh:
Japanese, 1 medium, 2½ ∞3½ 118
native, 1 medium, 1.1 oz. 32
Persimmon, dried, fuyu *(Frieda's)*, ⅓ cup, 1.4 oz. 140
Pesto sauce:
in jars *(Sonoma)*, ¼ cup 110
refrigerated *(Contadina* Reduced Fat), ¼ cup 230
refrigerated *(Di Giorno)*, ¼ cup 320
refrigerated, sun-dried tomato *(Contadina)*, ¼ cup 200
mix *(Knorr)*, ⅓ pkg. 15
mix, creamy *(Knorr)*, ⅕ pkg. 30
mix, sun-dried tomato *(Knorr)*, ⅓ pkg. 45
Picante sauce (see also "Salsa"), 2 tbsp.:
(Pace) 10
all varieties *(Chi-Chi's)* 10

Picante sauce *(cont.)*
all varieties *(Old El Paso)* 10
hot *(Sun-Vista)* 10
jalapeño, zesty, hot, medium, or mild *(Rosarita)* 10
mild *(Sun-Vista)* 5
Pickle, cucumber, 1 oz., except as noted:
bread and butter, chips *(Claussen),* 4 slices or 1 oz. 20
bread and butter, chips *(Vlasic)* 25
bread and butter, chunks *(Nalley* Banquet) 25
chips *(Nalley* Cucumber) 35
chips, w/honey *(Pickle Eater's)* 25
dill, all varieties *(Del Monte)* 5
dill, all varieties *(Vlasic)* 5
kosher, spears *(Hebrew National/Shorr's)* 4
sour *(Claussen* New York/Garlic Deli), ½ pickle 5
sour, kosher, garlic *(Hebrew National/Shorr's)* 3
sweet, all varieties *(Del Monte)* 40
sweet, all varieties *(Vlasic)* 40
sweet, gherkins or nubbins *(Nalley)* 25
Pickle relish, cucumber, 1 tbsp.:
hamburger *(Nalley)* 15
hamburger or sweet *(Del Monte)* 20
hot dog *(Del Monte)* 15
India *(Heinz)* 20
piccalilli, tomato *(Pickle Eater's)* 10
red hot *(Ron's)* 15
sweet *(Claussen)* 15
sweet *(Nalley)* 20
Pickling spice *(Tone's),* 1 tsp. 10
Pie, frozen:
apple *(Banquet),* ⅕ pie 300
apple *(Mrs. Smith's* 9), ⅛ pie 310
apple *(Mrs. Smith's* Dutch/Old Fashioned 9), ⅛ pie . . .350
apple-cranberry *(Mrs. Smith's),* ⅙ pie 280
banana cream *(Banquet),* ⅓ pie 350
banana cream *(Mrs. Smith's),* ¼ pie 280
banana cream *(Pet-Ritz),* ⅓ pie 350
berry or blackberry *(Mrs. Smith's),* ⅙ pie 280
blueberry *(Mrs. Smith's),* ⅙ pie 260
Boston creme, see "Cake, frozen"

cherry *(Banquet)*, ⅕ pie 290
cherry *(Mrs. Smith's* 9), ⅛ pie 310
cherry *(Mrs. Smith's* Old Fashioned 9), ⅛ pie 320
chocolate cream *(Banquet)*, ⅓ pie 360
chocolate cream *(Pet-Ritz)*, ⅓ pie 340
chocolate cream *(Sara Lee)*, ⅕ pie 500
coconut cream *(Banquet)*, ⅓ pie 350
coconut cream *(Pet-Ritz)*, ⅓ pie 350
coconut custard *(Mrs. Smith's)*, ⅕ pie 280
fudge vanilla cream *(Pet-Ritz)*, ⅓ pie 350
lemon cream *(Banquet)*, ⅓ pie 360
lemon meringue *(Sara Lee* Homestyle), ⅙ pie 350
mince/mincemeat *(Mrs. Smith's)*, ⅙ pie 300
peach *(Banquet)*, ⅕ pie 270
peach *(Mrs. Smith's* 9), ⅛ pie 310
pecan *(Mrs. Smith's* 10), ⅛ pie 500
pumpkin, hearty *(Mrs. Smith's* 9), ⅛ pie 240
pumpkin custard *(Mrs. Smith's* 9), ⅛ pie 240
raspberry or strawberry-rhubarb *(Mrs. Smith's)*, ⅙ pie . 280
strawberry *(Mrs. Smith's)*, ⅕ pie 280
Pie, mix, chocolate silk *(Jell-O)*, ⅙ pie* 310
Pie crust:
chocolate cookie *(Ready Crust)*, ⅛ crust 110
cookie crumbs *(Oreo)*, 2 tbsp. 80
graham *(Honey Maid)*, ⅙ crust 140
graham crumbs *(Honey Maid)*, 2 tbsp. 70
Pie crust, frozen or refrigerated, ⅛ crust:
(Pet-Ritz 9) 80
(Pet-Ritz Extra Large 9⅝) 110
(Pillsbury All Ready) 120
deep dish, all varieties *(Pet-Ritz)* 90
vegetable shortening *(Pet-Ritz)* 80
Pie crust mix *(Betty Crocker)*, ⅛ of 9 crust* 110
Pie filling, canned, ⅓ cup, except as noted:
apple *(Lucky Leaf/Lucky Leaf* Premium) 90
apple *(Musselman's* 24 oz.) 100
apple, blueberry, or cherry *(Lucky Leaf* Lite) 60
apricot or blackberry *(Lucky Leaf)* 90
blueberry *(Lucky Leaf/Musselman's)* 100
cherry *(Lucky Leaf/Musselman's)* 100

Pie filling *(cont.)*

cherry, dark sweet *(Lucky Leaf/Musselman's)* 110
cherry, red tart, in water *(Oregon)*, ⅔ cup 60
coconut creme *(Lucky Leaf)* 110
lemon *(Lucky Leaf/Musselman's 22/25 oz.)* 130
mince *(None Such)* 190
mince *(S&W)*, ¼ cup 180
mince, w/brandy and rum *(None Such)* 200
mince, condensed *(None Such)*, 4 tsp. 150
peach *(Lucky Leaf)* 80
pineapple *(Lucky Leaf/Musselman's)* 100
pumpkin *(Libby's* Mix), ½ cup 100
pumpkin *(Stokely)* 100
raisin *(Lucky Leaf)* 100
strawberry *(Lucky Leaf/Musselman's)* 80
strawberry-rhubarb *(Lucky Leaf)* 90
Pierogi, frozen or refrigerated:
potato cheese *(Empire* Kosher), 4 oz. 214
potato onion *(Empire* Kosher), 4 oz. 165
potato onion *(Giorgio)*, 3 pieces 230
Pigeon peas, ½ cup:
fresh, boiled, drained 86
canned, dried *(El Jib)* 80
canned, green *(Tupi)* 70
dried, boiled 102
Pignoli nut, see "Pine nut"
Pike, meat only:
northern, baked or broiled, 4 oz. 128
walleye, baked or broiled, 4 oz. 135
Pili nut, dried, shelled, 1 oz. 204
Pimiento, in jars, drained *(S&W)*, 2¼ oz. 20
Piña colada mixer, canned *(Goya)*, ⅓ cup 120
Pine nut, dried:
pignolia *(Frieda's)*, ¼ cup, 1.1 oz. 150
pignolia *(Krinos)*, .5 oz. 90
pignolia *(Progresso)*, 1-oz. jar 170
pinyon, 1 oz. 161
Pineapple:
fresh, diced, ½ cup 39
fresh, sliced *(Dole)*, 2 slices 90

canned, ½ cup, except as noted:

in juice, all varieties, except slices *(Del Monte)* 70
in juice, chunks or tidbits *(Dole)* 60
in juice, crushed *(Dole)* 70
in juice, slices *(Del Monte)*, 2 slices 60
in juice, slices *(Dole)*, 2 slices, 4 oz. 60
in light syrup, chunks, in jars *(Sunfresh)* 90
in light syrup, sliced *(Dole)*, 2 slices 90
in heavy syrup, crushed or chunks *(Del Monte)* 90
dried *(Sonoma)*, 1.4 oz. 140
Pineapple, candied *(Paradise/White Swan)*, 1 oz. . . .90
Pineapple drink *(Tropicana* Punch), 8 fl. oz. 120
Pineapple drink blends, 8 fl. oz.:
coconut *(Farmer's Market)* 120
coconut nectar *(Kern's)* 200
grapefruit, pink *(Dole)* 130
punch *(Tropicana Twister)* 130
Pineapple juice, 8 fl. oz.:
(Del Monte) 130
(S&W) 110
chilled *(Dole)* 130
Pineapple juice blends, 8 fl. oz.:
orange, orange-banana *(Dole)* 120
orange-strawberry *(Dole)* 130
Pineapple salsa *(Sorrell Ridge)*, 2 tbsp. 12
Pineapple topping, 2 tbsp.:
(Kraft) 110
(Smucker's) 110
Pink beans, ½ cup:
dried, boiled 125
canned *(Goya)* 120
canned, in tomato sauce *(Goya* Guisadas) 100
Pinquito beans, canned *(S&W)*, ½ cup 80
Pinto beans, ½ cup, except as noted:
dried *(Arrowhead Mills)*, ¼ cup 150
dried, boiled 117
canned *(Allens/East Texas Fair/Brown Beauty)* 110
canned *(Gebhardt)* 90
canned *(Green Giant/Joan of Arc)* 110
canned, w/bacon *(Trappey's/Trappey's* JalaPinto) 120

Pistachio nuts:
dried, in shell *(Dole)*, 1 oz. 90
dried, shelled *(Dole)*, 1 oz. 163
dry-roasted, in shell *(Planters)*, ½ cup, 1 oz. edible 160
Pita, see "Bread"
Pizza, frozen, 1 pie, except as noted:
bacon burger *(Totino's Party)*, ½ pie 380
Canadian bacon *(Jeno's Crisp 'N Tasty)* 430
Canadian bacon *(Totino's Party)*, ½ pie 320
cheese:
    (Celeste Large), ¼ pie 320
    (Jeno's Microwave for One) 240
    (Totino's Microwave for One) 240
    (Totino's Party), ½ pie 320
    (Totino's Party Family Size), ⅓ pie 360
    four *(Celeste* for One) 540
    four, zesty *(Celeste* Large), ¼ pie 330
    three *(Pappalo's* Deep Dish), ¼ pie 370
    three *(Pappalo's* Deep Dish for One) 540
    three *(Pappalo's* for One) 500
    three *(Pappalo's* Pizzaria Crust 9), ½ pie 400
    three *(Totino's* Select), ⅓ pie 300
    two, and Canadian bacon *(Totino's* Select), ⅓ pie . . . 310
    two, and pepperoni or sausage *(Totino's* Select),
      ⅓ pie 360
combination *(Jeno's* Microwave for One) 310
combination *(Jeno's Crisp 'N Tasty)* 520
combination *(Totino's* Microwave for One) 310
combination *(Totino's Party)*, ½ pie 390
combination or sausage *(Totino's Party* Family), ¼ pie . 300
hamburger or pepperoni *(Jeno's Crisp 'N Tasty)* 500
hamburger or zesty Mexican *(Totino's Party)*, ½ pie . . . 370
Italiano, zesty *(Totino's Party)*, ½ pie 390
w/meat *(Celeste* Suprema Large), ⅕ pie 290
meat, four *(Tombstone Special Order* 9), ⅓ pie 400
meat, four, or sausage *(Pappalo's* Deep Dish), ⅕ pie . . . 330
meat, three *(Jeno's Crisp 'N Tasty)* 500
meat, three *(Totino's Party)*, ½ pie 360
pepperoni *(Celeste* Large), ¼ pie 350
pepperoni *(Pappalo's* Deep Dish), ⅕ pie 340

pepperoni *(Pappalo's* Deep Dish for One) 540
pepperoni *(Pappalo's* for One) 520
pepperoni *(Tombstone* Original 9), ⅓ pie 340
pepperoni *(Tombstone For One)* 580
pepperoni *(Totino's Party* Family), ⅓ pie 410
pepperoni or sausage *(Totino's* Microwave for One) 280
pepperoni and sausage *(Pappalo's* Deep Dish), ⅕ pie . 340
pepperoni, sausage, or pepperoni and sausage
   (Pappalo's Pizzaria Crust 9), ½ pie 440
pepperoni, sausage, or supreme *(Totino's Party)*, ½ pie . 380
sausage *(Jeno's Crisp 'N Tasty)* 510
sausage *(Pappalo's* Pizzaria Crust 12), ¼ pie 380
sausage, Italian *(Tombstone For One)* 560
sausage, three *(Tombstone Special Order* 9), ⅓ pie . . . 390
sausage or pepperoni *(Jeno's* Microwave for One) 280
sausage and pepperoni:
   (Pappalo's Deep Dish for One) 550
   (Pappalo's for One) 530
   or supreme *(Totino's* Select), ⅓ pie 360
spinach feta *(Amy's)* 320
super *(Tombstone Special Order* 12), ⅙ pie 350
supreme *(Jeno's Crisp 'N Tasty)* 520
supreme *(Pappalo's* Deep Dish), ⅕ pie 350
supreme *(Pappalo's* Deep Dish for One) 540
supreme *(Pappalo's* for One) 520
supreme *(Pappalo's* Pizzaria Crust 12), ¼ pie 390
supreme *(Tombstone For One)* 570
supreme *(Totino's* Microwave for One) 290
vegetable *(Celeste* for One) 480
vegetable *(Tombstone For One* ½ Less Fat) 360
Pizza, bagel, mini, frozen, 4 pieces:
cheese, three *(Ore-Ida* Bagel Bits) 190
cheeseburger *(Ore-Ida* Bagel Bits) 210
supreme *(Ore-Ida* Bagel Bits) 180
Pizza, French bread, frozen:
cheese *(Healthy Choice),* 6 oz. 340
cheese *(Lean Cuisine),* 6 oz. 320
cheese *(Stouffer's),* ½ of 10⅜-oz. pkg. 360
cheeseburger *(Stouffer's),* ½ of 11⅞-oz. pkg. 420
deluxe *(Lean Cuisine),* 6⅛ oz. 320

Pizza, French bread *(cont.)*
deluxe *(Stouffer's)*, ½ of 12⅜-oz. pkg. 430
double cheese *(Stouffer's)*, ½ of 11¾-oz. pkg. 420
meat, three *(Stouffer's)*, ½ of 12½-oz. pkg. 460
pepperoni *(Healthy Choice)*, 6 oz. 340
pepperoni *(Lean Cuisine)*, 5¼ oz. 310
pepperoni *(Stouffer's)*, ½ of 11¼-oz. pkg. 440
sausage *(Healthy Choice)*, 6 oz. 320
sausage *(Stouffer's)*, ½ of 12-oz. pkg. 430
supreme *(Healthy Choice)*, 6.35 oz. 330
vegetable *(Healthy Choice)*, 6 oz. 280
vegetable, deluxe *(Stouffer's)*, ½ of 12¾-oz. pkg. 380
Pizza, Italian bread, frozen, 1 piece:
cheese, four *(Celeste)* 300
chicken, zesty *(Celeste)* 260
deluxe *(Celeste)* 290
pepperoni *(Celeste)* 320
Pizza crust, refrigerated *(Pillsbury)*, ¼ crust 180
Pizza crust mix*:
(Martha White), ¼ crust 170
deep pan *(Martha White)*, ⅕ crust 150
Pizza sandwich, frozen, 1 piece:
cheese *(Amy's Pocketfuls)* 290
deluxe *(Lean Pockets)* 270
meat, mega *(Totino's* Big & Hearty) 330
pepperoni *(Croissant Pockets)* 350
pepperoni *(Hot Pockets)* 350
pepperoni *(Totino's* Big & Hearty) 350
pepperoni style *(Amy's Pocketfuls)* 220
sausage or pepperoni and sausage *(Hot Pockets)* 340
vegetable *(Ken & Robert's Veggie Pockets)* 270
vegetable, pepperoni style *(Amy's)* 220
Pizza sauce, ¼ cup:
(Contadina) 25
(Contadina Chunky) 30
(Contadina Pizza Squeeze) 35
(Pastorelli Italian Chef) 40
(Prince Traditional) 20
(Progresso) 35
w/cheese, Italian *(Contadina)* 30

w/cheese, three *(Contadina* Chunky) 35
mushroom *(Contadina* Chunky) 30
pepperoni *(Contadina)* 30
Pizza snacks, 3 oz.:
cheese, double *(Hot Pockets* Pizza Snacks) 210
cheese, three *(Totino's* Pizza Rolls) 200
combination or spicy Italian *(Totino's* Pizza Rolls) 220
hamburger and cheese *(Totino's* Pizza Rolls) 200
meat, three *(Totino's* Pizza Rolls) 210
pepperoni *(Hot Pockets* Pizza Snacks) 220
pepperoni and cheese *(Totino's* Pizza Rolls) 230
pepperoni and sausage *(Hot Pockets* Pizza Snacks) 210
sausage *(Hot Pockets* Pizza Snacks) 200
sausage and cheese or supreme *(Totino's* Pizza Rolls) . 210
sausage and mushroom *(Totino's* Pizza Rolls) 200
Plantain:
raw, 1 medium, 9.7 oz. 218
cooked, sliced, ½ cup 89
fried *(Goya* Tostone), 3 pieces 170
Plum:
fresh *(Dole),* 2 plums 70
fresh, pitted, sliced, ½ cup 46
canned, in juice, 3 plums, 2 tbsp. liquid 55
canned, in light syrup, 3 plums, 2¾ tbsp. liquid 83
canned, in heavy syrup, 3 plums, 2¾ tbsp. liquid 119
canned, in heavy syrup, whole *(S&W),* ½ cup 130
canned, purple, in heavy syrup *(Oregon),* ½ cup 100
Plum sauce *(La Choy),* 1 tbsp. 25
Poke greens, canned *(Allens),* ½ cup 35
Polenta, refrigerated *(Frieda's),* 4 oz. 100
Polenta mix *(Fantastic Foods),* 1 cup* 260
Polish sausage (see also "Kielbasa"):
beef *(Hebrew National),* 4-oz. link 330
skinless *(John Morrell),* 2 oz. 180
Pollock, meat only:
Atlantic, baked or broiled, 4 oz. 134
walleye, baked or broiled, 4 oz. 128
Pomegranate, 1 medium, 9.7 oz. 104
Pomegranate juice *(R.W. Knudsen),* 8 fl. oz. 150
Pompano, meat only, baked or broiled, 4 oz. 239

Popcorn, unpopped, 2 tbsp., except as noted:
(Arrowhead Mills), ¼ cup, 1¾ oz. 180
(Healthy Choice Butter Flavor), 3 tbsp. 120
(Healthy Choice Natural Flavor), 3 tbsp. 120
(Orville Redenbacher Original/White/Hot Air) 90
(Redenbudders Movie Theater) 110
(Smart Pop Movie Theater) 90
microwave *(Smart Pop)* 100
microwave, caramel *(Orville Redenbacher)* 180
microwave, white or golden cheddar *(Smart Pop)* 170
microwave, zesty or herb and garlic *(Redenbudders)* . . . 180
Popcorn, popped:
(Barrel O'Fun Canola), 3 cups 145
(Barrel O'Fun Light), 3 cups 110
(Chester's Triple Mix), 1½ cups 140
air-popped *(Bachman* Lite), 5 cups 120
air-popped, white or yellow *(Jolly Time),* 5 cups 100
butter/butter flavor *(Chester's),* 3 cups 160
butter/butter flavor *(Smart Snackers),* .66-oz. bag 90
caramel *(Barrel O'Fun* Fat Free), ¾ cup 120
caramel *(Chester's),* ¾ cup 130
caramel *(Cracker Jack* Fat Free), 1 cup, 1 oz. 110
caramel, w/peanuts *(Barrel O'Fun),* ⅔ cup 130
caramel, w/peanuts *(Cracker Jack),* ⅔ cup 120
caramel, w/peanuts *(Old Dutch),* 1 oz. 128
cheddar *(Chester's),* 3 cups 190
cheddar, white *(Barrel O'Fun),* 3 cups 185
cheddar, white *(Chester's),* 3 cups 190
cheddar, white *(Smart Snackers),* .66-oz. bag 90
cheese *(Barrel O'Fun),* 2½ cups 135
cheese *(Barrel O'Fun* Low Fat), 2½ cups 140
microwave *(Jolly Time),* 4 cups 160
microwave *(Jolly Time* Light), 4 cups 100
microwave, butter *(Chester's),* 5 cups 200
microwave, butter flavor *(Jolly Time),* 4 cups 140
microwave, butter flavor *(Jolly Time* Light), 4 cups 80
toffee, butter *(Smart Snackers),* .9-oz. bag 110
toffee, w/nuts *(Franklin),* ⅔ cup 140
toffee, w/pecans and almonds *(Cracker Jack),* 1 oz. 130
toffee crunch *(Smartfood),* ¾ cup 130

Popcorn cakes:
all varieties, except caramel *(Orville Redenbacher* Mini),
　8 cakes 55
butter *(Orville Redenbacher),* 2 cakes 130
caramel *(Orville Redenbacher),* 1 cake 30
caramel *(Orville Redenbacher* Mini), 7 cakes 50
cheddar, white *(Lundberg* Mini), 5 cakes 70
cheddar, white *(Orville Redenbacher),* 2 cakes 60
Porgy, see "Scup"
Pork, meat only, 4 oz., except as noted:
leg, see "Ham"
loin, blade, broiled, lean w/fat 446
loin, blade, broiled, lean only 340
loin, blade, roasted, lean w/fat 413
loin, blade, roasted, lean only 316
loin, center, broiled, lean w/fat 358
loin, center, broiled, lean only 262
loin, center, roasted, lean w/fat 346
loin, center, roasted, lean only 272
loin, center rib, broiled, lean w/fat 389
loin, center rib, broiled, lean only 293
loin, center rib, roasted, lean w/fat 361
loin, center rib, roasted, lean only 278
loin, top, broiled, lean w/fat 408
loin, top, broiled, lean only 293
loin, top, roasted, lean only 278
shoulder, whole, roasted, lean w/fat 370
shoulder, whole, roasted, lean only 277
shoulder, arm (picnic), roasted, lean w/fat 375
shoulder, arm (picnic), roasted, lean only 259
shoulder, Boston blade, braised, lean w/fat 421
shoulder, Boston blade, braised, lean only 333
shoulder, Boston blade, broiled, lean w/fat 397
shoulder, Boston blade, broiled, lean only 311
shoulder, Boston blade, roasted, lean only 290
sirloin, broiled, lean w/fat 375
sirloin, broiled, lean only 276
sirloin, roasted, lean w/fat 330
sirloin, roasted, lean only 268

Pork *(cont.)*

sparibs, braised, lean w/fat, 6.3 oz. (1 lb. raw
  w/bone) 703
tenderloin, roasted, lean only 188
Pork, barbecued, refrigerated:
shredded *(Lloyd's),* ¼ cup 90
sparibs *(Lloyd's),* 3 ribs w/sauce 380
sparibs, baby back *(Lloyd's),* 3 ribs w/sauce 330
Pork, cured (see also "Ham"), 4 oz.:
arm (picnic), roasted, lean w/fat 318
arm (picnic), roasted, lean only 193
blade roll, lean w/fat, roasted 325
Pork, pickled:
hocks *(Hormel),* 2 oz. 110
tidbits *(Hormel),* 2 oz. 100
Pork, refrigerated, raw:
loin, center *(John Morrell Table Trim),* 4 oz. 190
smoked shoulder butt *(Oscar Mayer Sweet Morsel),*
  3 oz. 180
tenderloin *(John Morrell Table Trim),* 4 oz. 120
Pork dinner, frozen, boneless:
chop, country fried *(Marie Callender),* 15 oz. 550
patty, grilled glazed *(Healthy Choice),* 9.6 oz. 300
rib shape *(Swanson),* 1 pkg. 470
rib shape, barbecue sauce *(Swanson Hungry-Man),*
  1 pkg. 770
riblet *(Banquet* Extra Helping), 15.25 oz. 720
Pork entree, frozen:
cutlet *(Banquet),* 10¼ oz. 420
rib shape, barbecue sauce *(Swanson Lunch and More),*
  1 pkg. 370
riblet *(Banquet),* 10 oz. 400
Pork gravy, ¼ cup:
canned *(Franco-American Golden)* 45
canned *(Heinz Homestyle)* 25
mix* *(Durkee/French's)* 10
Pork lunch meat:
(Hormel Deli Pork Roast), 2 oz. 70
seasoned *(Boar's Head),* 2 oz. 80
Pork rind snack *(Old Dutch Bac'n Puffs),* ½ oz. 80

Pork seasoning mix, 1/8 pkg.:
(Shake'n Bake Original Recipe) 40
barbecue glaze *(Shake'n Bake)* 35
extra crispy *(Oven Fry)* 60
hot and spicy *(Shake'n Bake)* 45
Pot roast, see "Beef dinner" and "Beef entree"
Pot roast seasoning mix:
(Lawry's), 1 tsp. 5
sauerbraten *(Knorr)*, 1/6 pkg. 35
Potato:
raw *(Dole)*, 1 medium, 5.3 oz. 100
baked in skin, 1 medium, 4 3/4 ∞ 2 1/3 diam. 220
boiled in skin, peeled, 2 1/2 -diam. potato 119
boiled w/out skin, 1/2 cup 67
microwaved in skin, 1 medium, 4 3/4 ∞ 2 1/3 diam. 212
Potato, canned:
whole *(Butterfield/Sunshine)*, 5.6 oz., 2 1/2 pieces 90
whole *(Stokely/Stokely No Salt)*, 5 1/2 oz. 80
whole, new *(S&W)*, 1/2 cup 60
sliced *(Butterfield)*, 1/2 cup 100
sliced, new *(Del Monte)*, 2/3 cup 60
Potato, frozen (see also "Potato dishes, frozen"):
(Ore-Ida Deep Fries/Deep Fries Crinkle Cuts), 3 oz. 160
(Ore-Ida Shoestrings), 3 oz. 150
(Ore-Ida Steak Fries), 3 oz. 110
(Ore-Ida Crispers!), 3 oz. 220
(Ore-Ida Crispy Crowns!), 3 oz. 190
(Ore-Ida Crispy Crunchies!/Zesties), 3 oz. 160
(Ore-Ida Fast Fries/Waffle Fries), 3 oz. 150
(Ore-Ida Golden Crinkles), 3 oz. 140
(Ore-Ida Golden Fries), 3 oz. 120
cottage fries *(Ore-Ida)*, 3 oz. 130
country fries *(Ore-Ida)*, 3 oz. 120
hash brown *(Ore-Ida Microwave)*, 4-oz. pkg. 220
hash brown *(Ore-Ida Golden Patties)*, 1 piece 160
hash brown, Southern style *(Ore-Ida)*, 3/4 cup 80
hash brown, toaster *(Ore-Ida)*, 2 pieces 190
mashed *(Ore-Ida)*, 2/3 cup 90
O'Brien *(Ore-Ida)*, 3/4 cup 60
puffs *(Hot Tots)*, 3 oz. 160

Potato, frozen *(cont.)*
puffs *(Tater Tots)*, 3 oz. 160
Potato, mix, ½ cup*, except as noted:
(Betty Crocker Potato Buds), ⅔ cup* 160
all varieties (Betty Crocker Potato Shakers), ⅔ cup* . . . 140
all varieties, except sour cream and chive (Hungry Jack
    Casserole) 150
au gratin or julienne (Betty Crocker) 110
cheddar (Betty Crocker Homestyle) 120
cheddar, smokey, white, or bacon (Betty Crocker) 120
cheddar and bacon (Betty Crocker Twice Baked),
    ⅔ cup* 210
cheddar and sour cream (Betty Crocker), ⅔ cup* 130
cheese, three (Betty Crocker) 120
chicken and vegetable (Betty Crocker), ⅔ cup* 140
garlic, creamy (Betty Crocker), ⅔ cup* 150
hash browns (Betty Crocker) 200
herb garlic (Shake'n Bake Perfect Potatoes), ⅙ pkg. . . . 20
Italian, southern (Good Harvest), ⅓ cup 110
mashed:
    (Hungry Jack Flakes) 160
    (Pillsbury Idaho Flakes) 150
    (Pillsbury Idaho Granules) 160
    all flavors (Hungry Jack) 150
    butter and herb, roasted garlic, or sour cream–chive
        (Betty Crocker) 160
    sour cream–chive (Betty Crocker Potato Buds),
        ⅔ cup* 190
ranch or scalloped (Betty Crocker) 130
scalloped, cheesy (Betty Crocker Homestyle) 120
scalloped, and ham (Betty Crocker) 120
sour cream and chive (Betty Crocker) 120
sour cream and chive (Hungry Jack Casserole) 160
Potato, stuffed, see "Potato dishes, frozen"
Potato, sweet, see "Sweet potato"
Potato chips and crisps, 1 oz.:
(Lay's/Lay's Unsalted) 150
(Lay's Wavy/Wavy Ranch) 160
(Old Dutch/Old Dutch Ripl) 150
(Ruffles Reduced Fat) 140

(Wise Ripple) 150
all varieties *(Barbara's)*, 1¼ cups or 1 oz. 150
all varieties *(Lay's* Baked) 110
all varieties, except cheddar–sour cream *(Ruffles)* 150
baked, all varieties *(Lay's)* 110
barbecue *(Lay's* Hickory/*Lay's KC Masterpiece)* 150
barbecue *(Old Dutch/Old Dutch Ripl)* 150
barbecue, mesquite *(Old Dutch* Kettle) 130
cheddar–sour cream *(Barrel O'Fun* Ripple) 150
cheddar–sour cream *(Old Dutch)* 160
cheddar–sour cream *(Ruffles)* 160
hot *(Lay's* Flamin') 150
jalapeño *(Krunchers!)* 140
jalapeño-cheddar *(Old Dutch)* 130
onion, French *(Old Dutch* Ripl) 150
onion-garlic *(Barrel O'Fun)* 140
onion-garlic *(Old Dutch)* 140
pizza *(Lay's)* 160
salsa-cheese *(Lay's)* 160
salt and sour *(Barrel O'Fun)* 150
salt and vinegar *(Lay's)* 160
salt and vinegar *(Old Dutch)* 130
sour cream and onion *(Lay's)* 160
sour cream and onion *(Ruffle's* Reduced Fat) 130
sour cream–onion *(Old Dutch)* 150
Potato dishes, canned, 7.5 oz.:
scalloped, and ham *(Hormel)* 260
sliced, and beef *(Dinty Moore)* 230
Potato dishes, frozen:
au gratin *(Stouffer's* Side Dish), 4.6 oz. 130
au gratin, w/ham, broccoli *(Banquet* Family), ⅔ cup . . . 210
baked, broccoli-cheese *(Ore-Ida* Twice Baked), 5 oz. . . . 150
baked, broccoli-cheese *(Weight Watchers)*, 10 oz. 250
baked, butter flavor *(Ore-Ida* Twice Baked), 5 oz. 200
baked, cheddar *(Ore-Ida* Twice Baked), 5 oz. 190
baked, sour cream–chive *(Ore-Ida* Twice Baked), 5 oz. . 200
cheddar *(Lean Cuisine* Deluxe), 1 pkg. 230
cheddar-broccoli *(Healthy Choice)*, 1 pkg., 10.5 oz. 330
garden casserole *(Healthy Choice)*, 1 pkg., 9.25 oz. 210
scalloped *(Stouffer's* Side Dish), 4.6 oz. 140

Potato dishes, frozen *(cont.)*

wedges, topped w/Swiss cheese, chicken, mushroom
  (Marie Callender), 13 oz. 390
wedges, topped w/Swiss cheese, ham, broccoli *(Marie
  Callender)*, 13 oz. 380
Potato pancake, frozen:
(Empire Kosher), 2-oz. cake 80
mini *(Empire* Kosher), 2 cakes, 2 oz. 90
Potato pancake mix *(Hungry Jack)*, 3 cakes*, 3 90
Potato sticks:
(Butterfield), 1 cup 250
(French's), ¾ cup 180
(Pik-Nik Fabulous Fries), 1 oz. 150
hot *(Chester's* Fries Flamin'), 1 oz. 140
ketchup or shoestring *(Pik-Nik)*, ⅔ cup 160
Poultry, see specific listings
Pout, ocean, meat only, baked or broiled, 4 oz. 116
Preserves, see "Jam and preserves"
Pretzels:
(Barrel O'Fun Minis), 1 oz. 105
(Mister Salty Mini), 1 oz. 110
(Old Dutch), 1⅛-oz. bag 125
(Quinlan Nuggets), 1.1-oz. bag 130
(Quinlan Party Thins/Sticks) 1 oz. 110
Bavarian *(Rold Gold)*, 1 oz. 110
chips *(Mister Salty)*, 1 oz. 110
Dutch *(Mister Salty)*, 2 pieces, 1.1 oz. 120
honey mustard–onion *(Old Dutch)*, 1.1 oz. 140
rods *(Old Dutch)*, 3 pieces, 1.2 oz. 130
rods *(Rold Gold)*, 1 oz. 110
sourdough, hard *(Rold Gold)*, 1 oz. 110
sticks *(Old Dutch)*, 1 oz. 110
sticks *(Rold Gold* Fat Free), 1 oz. 110
thins *(Quinlan)*, 1 oz. 120
thins *(Rold Gold/Rold Gold* Fat Free), 1 oz. 110
twists *(Old Dutch)*, 1 oz. 110
twists *(Mister Salty)*, 1 oz. 110
twists *(Rold Gold* Crispy Butter or Original), 1 oz. 110
twists, tiny *(Rold Gold* Fat Free), 1 oz. 100
Pretzel dip, cheddar-mustard *(Heluva* Good), ¼ cup . . . 100

Prickly pear *(Frieda's* Cactus Pear), 5 oz. 60
Prosciutto *(Primissimo)*, 2 oz. 210
Prune:
canned, in syrup, 5 medium and 2 tbsp. liquid 90
dried *(Del Monte)*, ¼ cup 120
dried *(Sunsweet)*, 6–8 pieces 100
dried, pitted *(Sonoma)*, ¼ cup 120
Prune juice, all varieties *(Del Monte)*, 8 fl. oz. 170
Pudding, 4 oz., except as noted:
banana *(Del Monte* Snack), 3.5-oz. cup 120
banana *(Hunt's Snack Pack)*, 3.5-oz. cup 120
butterscotch *(Hunt's Snack Pack)*, 3.5-oz. cup 130
butterscotch *(Swiss Miss)* 160
chocolate *(Hunt's Snack Pack)*, 3.5-oz. cup 145
chocolate, milk *(Hunt's Snack Pack)*, 3.5-oz. cup 145
chocolate almond *(Healthy Choice* Low Fat) 110
chocolate fudge *(Swiss Miss)* 175
chocolate fudge, double *(Healthy Choice* Low Fat) 110
chocolate marshmallow *(Hunt's Snack Pack)*,
  3.5-oz. cup 135
chocolate raspberry *(Healthy Choice* Low Fat) 110
chocolate swirl, caramel or peanut butter *(Hunt's Snack
  Pack)*, 3.5-oz. cup 145
chocolate swirl, caramel or vanilla *(Swiss Miss)* 170
lemon *(Hunt's Snack Pack)*, 3.5-oz. cup 125
tapioca *(Healthy Choice* Low Fat) 110
tapioca *(Hunt's Snack Pack)*, 3.5-oz. cup 125
tapioca *(Swiss Miss)* 140
vanilla *(Hunt's Snack Pack)*, 3.5-oz. cup 135
vanilla *(Swiss Miss)* 160
vanilla, French *(Healthy Choice* Low Fat) 110
vanilla-chocolate parfait *(Swiss Miss)* 165
vanilla-chocolate swirl *(Jell-O* Snack) 170
Pudding, mix, ½ cup*:
banana cream *(Jell-O)* 140
banana cream or butterscotch *(Jell-O* Instant) 150
butterscotch *(Jell-O)* 160
chocolate or chocolate fudge *(Jell-O)* 150
chocolate or chocolate fudge *(Jell-O* Instant) 160
coconut cream *(Jell-O)* 150

Pudding, mix *(cont.)*

coconut cream *(Jell-O Instant)* 160
custard *(Jell-O Americana)* 140
custard, tropical *(Goya Tembleque)* 100
flan *(Goya)* 100
flan *(Jell-O)* 140
flan, w/caramel *(Goya)* 190
lemon *(Jell-O)* 140
lemon *(Jell-O Instant)* 150
pistachio *(Jell-O Instant)* 160
tapioca *(Jell-O Americana)* 140
vanilla *(Jell-O)* 140
vanilla *(Jell-O Instant)* 160
vanilla, French *(Jell-O Instant)* 150
Pudding, rice, see "Rice pudding"
Pummelo, 1 medium, 5½ diam. 228
Pumpkin:
fresh, pulp, boiled, drained, mashed, ½ cup 24
canned *(Stokely)*, ½ cup 50
pie mix, see "Pie filling"
Pumpkin seeds:
roasted, in shell, 1 oz. or 85 seeds 127
dried, shelled, 1 oz. or 142 kernels 154
tamari-roasted, spicy *(Eden)*, 1 oz. 170
Purslane, boiled, drained, ½ cup 10
Quail, raw:
meat w/skin, 1 quail, 3.8 oz. (4.3 oz. w/bone) 210
meat only, 1 quail, 3.2 oz. (4.3 oz. w/bone and skin) . . . 123
Quince, pineapple, pulp *(Frieda's)*, 3.5 oz. 57
Quinoa:
dry *(Eden)*, ¼ cup 170
black and white *(Frieda's)*, 2 oz. dry or ½ cup cooked . 218
Quinoa seeds *(Arrowhead Mills)*, ¼ cup 140

R

Rabbit, domesticated, meat only:
roasted, 4 oz. 223
stewed, 4 oz. 234
stewed, diced, 1 cup 288
Radicchio, fresh, shredded *(Frieda's),* 2 cups, 3 oz. 20
Radish, 10 medium, ³/₄ −1 diam. 7
Radish, Oriental, raw:
(Frieda's Daikon), ²/₃ cup, 3 oz. 15
(Frieda's Lo Bok), ²/₃ cup, 3 oz. 40
1 medium, 7 ∞2¹/₄ diam. 62
Radish, white-icicle, 1 medium, .6 oz. 2
Rainbow baking morsels *(Nestlé),* 1 tbsp. 70
Raisin, seedless:
(Del Monte/Del Monte Golden), ¹/₄ cup 120
(Sun•Maid), ¹/₄ cup 130
monukka/Thompson *(Sonoma),* ¹/₄ cup 130
Raisin sauce *(Reese),* ¹/₄ cup 150
Ranch dip, 2 tbsp.:
(Heluva Good Classic) 60
(Marie's Creamy) 190
(Marie's Homestyle) 150
(Nalley) 110
(Old Dutch) 50
(Ruffles) 70
(Ruffles Low Fat) 40
bacon *(Marie's)* 150
peppercorn *(Marie's* Fat Free) 35
Ranch dip mix, cracked pepper *(Knorr),* ¹/₂ tsp. 5
Rapini, see "Broccoli rabe"
Raspberry:
fresh, ¹/₂ cup 31
canned, red, in heavy syrup *(Oregon),* ¹/₂ cup 120
frozen, red *(Big Valley),* ²/₃ cup 60

Raspberry drink, 8 fl. oz.:
hibiscus *(R.W. Knudsen)* 90
lemon *(Santa Cruz)* 120
Raspberry juice, 8 fl. oz.:
blend *(Dole* Country) 140
peach *(R.W. Knudsen)* 120
Raspberry nectar, frozen* *(R.W. Knudsen)*, 8 fl. oz. . . . 120
Rattlesnake beans, dried *(Frieda's)*, ½ cup 120
Ravioli, frozen or refrigerated:
cheese *(Amy's)*, 9.5 oz. 340
cheese *(Contadina* Family Pack/Four), 1 cup 290
cheese, four *(Contadina* Light), 1 cup 240
cheese, herb, Italian *(Di Giorno)*, 1 cup 350
cheese and garlic *(Di Giorno* Light), 1 cup 270
chicken, rosemary *(Contadina)*, 1¼ cups 330
chicken and rosemary *(Real Torino)*, 1 cup 300
crab, snow *(Monterey Pasta Company)*, 3 oz. 230
garden vegetable *(Contadina* Light), 1 cup 250
Gorgonzola *(Contadina)*, 1¼ cups 360
w/Italian sausage *(Di Giorno)*, ¾ cup 340
spinach and ricotta *(Real Torino)*, 1 cup 310
tomato and cheese *(Di Giorno* Light), 1 cup 280
Ravioli entree, canned, 1 cup, except as noted:
beef *(Libby's)*, 7¾ oz. 230
beef *(Progresso)* 260
beef, and meat sauce *(Hunt's* Homestyle) 220
beef, in meat sauce *(Franco-American* Superiore) 280
beef, mini, w/meat *(Chef Boyardee* Bowl), 7½ oz. 180
beef, w/pasta in tomato-cheese sauce *(Franco-
American)* 230
cheese *(Chef Boyardee)* 210
cheese *(Progresso)* 220
cheese, w/meat *(Chef Boyardee* Bowl), 7½ oz. 190
tomato sauce *(Hormel* Micro Cup), 7½ oz. 270
Ravioli entree, frozen, cheese:
(Lean Cuisine), 8.5 oz. 240
(Stouffer's), 10⅝ oz. 380
parmigiana *(Healthy Choice)*, 9 oz. 260
Red beans (see also "Kidney beans"), canned, ½ cup:
(Allens) 160

(Stokely) 110
(Van Camp) 90
small *(Hunt's)* 90
Red snapper, see "Snapper"
Refried beans, canned, ½ cup:
(Allens) 150
(Chi-Chi's) 130
(Gebhardt) 110
(Gebhardt No Fat) 90
(Las Palmas) 110
(Old El Paso) 110
(Rosarita) 110
(Rosarita No Fat) 120
all varieties *(Old El Paso/Las Palmas* Fat Free) 100
bacon *(Rosarita)* 115
black beans *(Old El Paso/Las Palmas)* 110
black beans *(Rosarito* Low Fat) 105
w/cheese *(Old El Paso)* 130
w/cheese, nacho, or green chilies *(Rosarita)* 110
w/green chilies *(Old El Paso)* 100
w/green chilies and lime *(Rosarita* No Fat) 100
w/jalapeño *(Gebhardt)* 105
w/salsa, zesty *(Rosarita* No Fat) 105
w/sausage *(Old El Paso)* 200
spicy *(Rosarita)* 120
vegetarian *(Chi-Chi's)* 80
vegetarian *(Gebhardt)* 120
vegetarian *(Old El Paso)* 100
Relish, see "Pickle relish" and specific listings
Remoulade sauce *(Zararain's)*, ¼ cup 80
Rennet *(Junket)*, 1 tablet 1
Rhubarb:
fresh *(Frieda's)*, ⅔ cup, 3 oz. 20
canned, in extra heavy syrup *(Oregon)*, ½ cup 180
frozen *(Stilwell)*, 1 cup 30
Rice (see also "Wild rice"), ¼ cup dry, except as
    noted:
arborio *(Fantastic Foods)* 210
basmati, brown *(Arrowhead Mills)* 150
basmati, brown *(Fantastic Foods)* 170

Rice *(cont.)*
basmati, white *(Fantastic Foods)* 180
brown *(Carolina/Mahatma/River)* 150
brown *(Success)*, ½ cup 150
brown, long grain *(S&W)* 150
brown, long grain *(Uncle Ben's* Whole Grain) 170
brown, precooked *(S&W* Quick), ½ cup 150
brown, quick or sweet *(Lundberg)* 150
glutinous or sweet *(Goya* Fancy Blue Rose/Valencia) . . . 170
jasmine *(Fantastic Foods)* 170
white *(Success)*, ½ cup 190
white, long grain *(Carolina)* 150
white, long grain *(Martha White)* 170
white, long grain *(River/Water Maid)* 160
white, long grain, instant *(Minute)*, ½ cup 170
white, long grain, parboiled *(Uncle Ben's Converted)* . . . 170
Rice cake, plain *(Quaker* Salted/Salt Free), 1 cake 35
Rice dishes, canned, 1 cup, except as noted:
Chinese fried *(La Choy)* 240
Spanish *(Old El Paso)* 130
Spanish *(Van Camp)*, ½ cup 90
Rice dishes, mix, 1 cup*, except as noted:
(Lipton Rice & Sauce Original Recipe) 280
and beans, Cajun *(Lipton* Rice & Sauce) 310
and beans, red *(Rice-A-Roni)* 280
beef *(Lipton* Rice & Sauce) 270
beef *(Rice-A-Roni)* 320
beef and mushroom *(Rice-A-Roni)* 290
broccoli Alfredo *(Lipton* Rice & Sauce) 320
broccoli au gratin *(Rice-A-Roni)* 370
broccoli au gratin *(Savory Classics)* 390
Cajun *(Lipton* Rice & Sauce) 270
cheddar, white, w/herbs *(Rice-A-Roni)* 340
cheddar broccoli *(Lipton* Rice & Sauce) 280
chicken *(Lipton* Rice & Sauce) 280
chicken *(Rice-A-Roni)* 310
chicken *(Rice-A-Roni* Less Salt) 280
chicken *(Savory Classics)* 300
chicken, creamy *(Lipton* Rice & Sauce) 290
chicken, roasted or Southwestern *(Lipton* Seasoned) . . . 260

chicken and broccoli *(Lipton* Rice & Sauce) 280
chicken and broccoli *(Rice-A-Roni)* 290
chicken and mushrooms *(Rice-A-Roni)* 360
chicken w/vegetables *(Rice-A-Roni)* 290
chicken and wild rice, almond *(Savory Classics)* 310
curry *(Lundberg One Step),* 2 oz. 160
fried *(Chun King),* ½ cup 125
fried *(Rice-A-Roni)* 320
fried *(Rice-A-Roni* Less Salt) 260
gumbo *(Mahatma)* 160
herb and butter *(Lipton* Rice & Sauce) 280
herb and butter *(Rice-A-Roni)* 310
long grain and wild *(Rice-A-Roni)* 240
long grain and wild, chicken-almonds *(Rice-A-Roni)* . . . 290
long grain and wild, pilaf *(Rice-A-Roni)* 240
medley *(Lipton* Rice & Sauce) 270
Mexican *(Savory Classics* Fiesta) 310
Mexican, cheesy *(Old El Paso)* 420
mushroom *(Lipton* Rice & Sauce) 270
mushroom and herb *(Lipton* Rice & Sauce) 290
Oriental *(Rice-A-Roni/Rice-A-Roni* Less Salt) 290
Oriental *(Savory Classics)* 290
Oriental, stir-fry *(Lipton* Seasoned Rice) 270
pilaf *(Lipton* Rice & Sauce) 260
pilaf *(Rice-A-Roni)* 310
pilaf, garden *(Savory Classics)* 240
risotto, all varieties *(Lundberg),* ¼ pkg. 140
risotto, chicken-Parmesan *(Lipton* Rice & Sauce) 270
salsa style *(Lipton* Seasoned Rice) 220
scampi style *(Lipton* Rice & Sauce) 270
Spanish *(Lipton* Rice & Sauce) 270
Spanish *(Rice-A-Roni)* 270
Spanish pilaf *(Knorr),* ⅓ cup 230
Spanish pilaf, brown *(Lundberg* Quick Fiesta) 190
sticky, w/coconut milk *(Thai Kitchen),* ½ cup* 240
Stroganoff *(Rice-A-Roni)* 360
teriyaki *(Lipton* Rice & Sauce) 270
yellow *(Goya),* 2 oz. 170
yellow, saffron *(Carolina/Mahatma),* 2 oz. 190

Rice flour, ¼ cup:
brown *(Arrowhead Mills)* 120
white *(Arrowhead Mills)* 160
Rice pudding:
canned *(Thank You)*, ½ cup 160
mix *(Goya)*, ½ cup* 90
mix *(Jell-O Americana)*, ½ cup* 160
Rice seasoning mix:
fried *(Durkee)*, ¼ pkg. 15
Mexican *(Lawry's)*, 1½ tbsp. 40
Rice-vegetable dishes, frozen, 10-oz. pkg.:
(Green Giant Medley) 240
and broccoli *(Green Giant)* 320
pilaf *(Green Giant)* 230
white and wild rice *(Green Giant)* 250
Rigatoni, refrigerated *(Tutta Pasta)*, 1 cup 290
Rigatoni dishes, canned, Italian garden sauce *(Hunt's*
Homestyle)*, 1 cup 165
Rigatoni entree, frozen, creamy, w/broccoli and
chicken *(Smart Ones)*, 9 oz. 230
Rockfish, meat only, baked or broiled, 4 oz. 137
Roe (see also "Caviar"):
raw, 1 oz. 40
baked, broiled, or microwaved, 4 oz. 231
Roll (see also "Croissant"), 1 roll, except as noted:
brown and serve *(Pepperidge Farm Hearth)*, 3 rolls 150
brown and serve, club *(Pepperidge Farm)* 120
brown and serve, French *(Pepperidge Farm 3)* 240
brown and serve, sourdough *(Arnold Francisco)* 80
crescent, butter *(Pepperidge Farm Heat & Serve)* 110
dill and onion *(Awrey's Deli Rounds)* 150
dinner *(Arnold August Bros.)* 90
dinner *(Brownberry Francisco Intl.)* 120
dinner *(Pepperidge Farm Country Style/Finger/Parker*
House/Poppy/Sesame)*, 3 rolls 150
dinner, all varieties *(Awrey's)*, 2 rolls, 1.6 oz. 110
dinner, potato *(Arnold)*, 2 rolls 110
dinner, potato *(Pepperidge Farm Deli Classic)* 80
dinner, sesame seed *(Arnold)*, 2 rolls 110
dinner, wheat *(Arnold August Bros.)* 100

egg, twist *(Arnold Levy* Old Country) 170
French, regular *(Pepperidge Farm)* 100
French, 7 grain *(Pepperidge Farm* 9) 80
French, sourdough *(Pepperidge Farm)* 100
garlic and pepper *(Awrey's* Deli Rounds) 150
golden twist *(Pepperidge Farm* Heat & Serve) 110
hamburger *(Pepperidge Farm)* 130
hamburger *(Roman Meal)* 120
hamburger *(Wonder)* 110
hamburger *(Wonder* 4) 130
hoagie (see also "sub," below) *(Awrey's)* 230
hot dog *(Pepperidge Farm)* 140
hot dog *(Roman Meal)* 110
hot dog *(Wonder)* 110
hot dog, Dijon *(Pepperidge Farm)* 140
kaiser *(Arnold Francisco* 6 /*Arnold Levy* Old Country) . 170
kaiser *(Awrey's)* 190
onion *(Arnold August Bros./Arnold Levy* Old Country) . 160
party *(Pepperidge Farm* 20), 5 rolls 170
sandwich *(Pepperidge Farm* Hearty) 230
sandwich *(Roman Meal)* 185
sandwich, multigrain or onion *(Pepperidge Farm)* 150
sandwich, potato *(Pepperidge Farm)* 160
sandwich, sesame seed *(Pepperidge Farm)* 140
sub *(Arnold Levy* Old Country) 140
Roll, frozen or refrigerated:
(Rich's Homestyle), 2 rolls 150
crescent *(Pillsbury* Reduced Fat), 1 roll 100
crescent, regular or cheese *(Pillsbury)*, 1 roll 110
dinner, wheat or white *(Pillsbury)*, 1 roll 110
Roll, mix, hot *(Pillsbury)*, 1/15 pkg.* 130
Roll, sweet, see "Bun, sweet"
Roman beans, dry *(Goya)*, 1/4 cup 80
Roselle, 1 oz. or 1/2 cup 14
Rosemary, dried, 1 tsp. 4
Rotini dishes, mix:
and cheese, w/broccoli *(Velveeta)*, 4 1/2 oz. 400
and cheese, three *(Lipton* Pasta & Sauce), 1 cup* 320
mushroom sauce *(Knorr)*, 2/3 cup 250
primavera *(Lipton* Pasta & Sauce), 1 cup* 320

Roughy, orange, meat only, baked or broiled, 4 oz. . . . 101
Roy Rogers, 1 serving:
breakfast items:

    bagel, plain or cinnamon raisin 300
    Big Country Breakfast Platter w/bacon 740
    Big Country Breakfast Platter w/ham 710
    Big Country Breakfast Platter w/sausage 920
    biscuit, plain 390
    biscuit, bacon 420
    biscuit, bacon and egg 470
    biscuit, *Cinnamon 'N' Raisin* 370
    biscuit, ham and cheese 450
    biscuit, ham and egg 460
    biscuit, ham, egg, and cheese 500
    biscuit, sausage 510
    biscuit, sausage and egg 560
    hash rounds 230
    orange juice 140
    pancakes, 3 pieces, plain 280
    pancakes, 3 pieces, w/2 strips bacon 350
    pancakes, 3 pieces, w/1 sausage 430
    sourdough sandwich, ham, egg, and cheese 480
sandwiches:
    bacon cheeseburger 490
    bacon cheeseburger, sourdough 730
    cheeseburger 300
    cheeseburger, ¼ lb. 470
    chicken, grilled 340
    chicken, grilled, sourdough 500
    chicken fillet 500
    Fisherman's Fillet, seasonal 490
    hamburger 260
    hamburger, ¼ lb. 430
    roast beef 260
chicken, fried:
    breast 370
    leg 170
    thigh 330
    wing 200

¼ Roy's Roaster:
    dark meat 490
    dark meat, w/skin off 190
    white meat 500
    white meat, w/skin off 190
chicken nuggets, 6 pieces 290
chicken nuggets, 9 pieces 460
salads:
    chicken, grilled 120
    garden 190
    side salad 140
potatoes:
    baked 130
    baked, w/margarine 240
    baked, w/margarine and sour cream 300
    fries, regular 350
    fries, large 430
    mashed, 5 oz. 92
    gravy for mashed potatoes 20
sides:
    baked beans, 5 oz. 160
    coleslaw, 5 oz. 295
    corn bread 310
vanilla frozen yogurt cone 180
Rutabaga, ½ cup:
fresh, boiled, drained, mashed 47
canned, diced *(Sunshine)* 30
Rye, whole-grain *(Arrowhead Mills)*, ¼ cup 160
Rye flakes, rolled *(Arrowhead Mills)*, ⅓ cup 110
Rye flour, medium *(Pillsbury)*, ¼ cup 100
Rye-wheat flour *(Pillsbury* Bohemian Style)*, ¼ cup 100

FOOD AND MEASURE	CALORIES

Sablefish, meat only:
baked, broiled, or microwaved, 4 oz. 284
smoked, 4 oz. 291
Saffron, 1 tsp. 2
Sage *(McCormick),* ¼ tsp. 1
Salad, complete, w/dressing, 3.5 oz., except as noted:
all varieties, except herb ranch *(Dole* Low Fat) 60
Caesar *(Dole)* 170
Caesar *(Dole Lunch for One),* 5.75 oz. 290
Caesar *(Dole Lunch for One* Low Fat), 5.75 oz. 120
Italian *(Dole Lunch for One* Low Fat), 7 oz. 130
Oriental *(Dole)* 120
ranch, classic *(Dole Lunch for One),* 7 oz. 260
ranch, herb *(Dole* Low Fat) 50
Romano *(Dole)* 150
spinach-bacon or sunflower ranch *(Dole)* 160
Salad dressing, 2 tbsp.:
balsamic vinegar *(S&W* Vintage) 35
berry vinaigrette *(Knott's Berry Farm)* 40
blue cheese *(Hellmann's)* 140
blue cheese *(Kraft Roka)* 90
blue cheese, chunky *(Marie's)* 180
blue cheese, chunky *(Wish-Bone)* 170
blue cheese, chunky *(Wish-Bone* Lite) 70
Caesar *(Cardini's* Original) 160
Caesar *(Hidden Valley Ranch* Fat Free) 30
Caesar *(Kraft* Classic) 110
Caesar *(Wish-Bone)* 110
Caesar creamy *(Hellmann's)* 170
Caesar creamy *(Wish-Bone)* 180
citrus vinaigrette *(Knott's Berry Farm)* 40
coleslaw *(Marie's)* 150
dill, creamy *(Nasoya Vegi-Dressing)* 60

Salad dressing *(cont.)*

French *(Kraft Catalina)* 140
French *(Wish-Bone Deluxe)* 120
French *(Wish-Bone Lite)* 50
French, honey and bacon *(Hidden Valley Ranch)* 150
French, sweet 'n spicy *(Wish-Bone)* 140
French, tangy *(Marie's)* 130
garlic, creamy *(Wish-Bone Fat Free)* 40
garlic, roasted, creamy *(Wish-Bone)* 110
garlic, zesty *(Cardini's)* 120
herb, garden *(Nasoya Vegi-Dressing)* 60
herb, Italian, and cheese *(Hidden Valley Ranch* Fat
  Free*)* 30
herb vinaigrette, zesty *(Marie's Fat Free)* 30
herbs and spices *(Seven Seas)* 120
honey Dijon *(Wish-Bone Fat Free)* 45
honey Dijon vinaigrette, zesty *(Marie's Fat Free)* 50
honey mustard *(Marie's)* 160
honey mustard *(Nalley)* 130
Italian *(Seven Seas Viva)* 110
Italian *(Wish-Bone)* 80
Italian *(Wish-Bone Classic House)* 140
Italian *(Wish-Bone Rubusto)* 90
Italian, 2 cheese *(Seven Seas)* 70
Italian, creamy *(Seven Seas)* 110
Italian, creamy *(Wish-Bone)* 110
Italian, garlic, creamy *(Marie's)* 180
Italian, herb and garlic, creamy *(Bernstein's)* 130
Italian, olive oil *(Wish-Bone Classic)* 70
Italian, Parmesan *(Hidden Valley Ranch Fat Free)* 20
mango–key lime vinegar *(S&W Vintage Lite)* 30
mayonnaise type, see "Mayonnaise"
olive oil vinaigrette *(Wish-Bone)* 60
Oriental rice wine vinegar *(S&W Vintage Lite)* 30
(Ott's Famous Original) 80
Parmesan, creamy *(Marie's Low Fat)* 35
Parmesan and onion *(Wish-Bone)* 110
peppercorn, ground *(Knott's Berry Farm)* 160
pesto *(Cardini's Pasta)* 140
poppy seed *(Marie's)* 150

potato salad *(Best Foods/Hellmann's One Step)* 160
ranch *(Hidden Valley Reduced Calorie)* 80
ranch *(Hidden Valley Ranch Original)* 140
ranch *(Seven Seas)* 150
ranch *(Wish-Bone)* 160
ranch, w/bacon *(Hidden Valley Ranch Original)* 150
ranch, buttermilk *(Marie's)* 180
ranch, creamy *(Marie's Reduced Calorie)* 100
ranch, Parmesan *(Marie's)* 180
ranch, zesty *(Marie's Low Fat)* 30
raspberry blush vinegar *(S&W Vintage Lite)* 40
raspberry vinaigrette, zesty *(Marie's Fat Free)* 35
red wine vinaigrette *(Wish-Bone)* 80
red wine vinegar *(Seven Seas Free)* 15
red wine vinegar, w/herbs *(S&W Vintage Lite)* 40
red wine vinegar and oil *(Seven Seas)* 110
Russian *(Seven Seas Viva)* 150
Russian *(Wish-Bone)* 110
sesame garlic *(Nasoya Vegi-Dressing)* 60
sour cream and dill *(Marie's)* 190
Thousand Island *(Marie's)* 240
Thousand Island *(Marie's Salad Bar)* 170
Thousand Island *(Nalley)* 120
Thousand Island *(Wish-Bone)* 140
Thousand Island, w/bacon *(Kraft)* 120
tomato, sun-dried, vinaigrette *(Knott's Berry Farm)* 100
tuna salad *(Best Foods/Hellmann's One Step)* 140
white wine vinaigrette, zesty *(Marie's Fat Free)* 40
Salad dressing mix, 2 tbsp.*:
buttermilk, farm, or ranch *(Good Seasons)* 120
Caesar, gourmet, or honey mustard *(Good Seasons)* . . . 150
cheese garlic or garlic and herbs *(Good Seasons)* 140
Italian *(Good Seasons Reduced Calorie)* 50
Italian, mild *(Good Seasons)* 150
Italian, regular or zesty *(Good Seasons)* 140
Mexican spice *(Good Seasons)* 140
Oriental sesame *(Good Seasons)* 150
Salad toppers *(McCormick Salad Toppin's)*, 1 1/3 tbsp. . . 35
Salami:
beef *(Hebrew National)*, 2 oz. 170

Salami *(cont.)*

beef *(Hebrew National* Reduced Fat), 2 oz. 110
beef *(Oscar Mayer* Machiach), 2 slices, 1.6 oz. 120
beer *(Oscar Mayer)*, 2 slices, 1.6 oz. 110
cooked *(Boar's Head)*, 2 oz. 130
cotto *(Oscar Mayer)*, 2 slices, 1.6 oz. 110
cotto, beef *(Oscar Mayer)*, 2 slices, 1.6 oz. 90
dry or hard *(Boar's Head)*, 1 oz. 110
dry or hard *(Hormel Homeland/Sandwich Maker)*, 1 oz. . 110
Genoa *(Di Lusso)*, 1 oz. 120
Genoa *(San Remo Brand)*, 1 oz. 120
hard *(Oscar Mayer)*, 3 slices, 1 oz. 100
"Salami," vegetarian, frozen *(Worthington)*, 3 slices . 130
Salmon, meat only, 4 oz.:
Atlantic, farmed, baked or broiled 234
Atlantic, wild, baked or broiled 206
chinook, baked or broiled 262
chum, baked or broiled 175
coho, farmed, baked or broiled 202
coho, wild, baked or broiled 158
coho, wild, boiled, poached, or steamed 209
pink, baked or broiled 169
sockeye, baked or broiled 245
Salmon, canned, ¼ cup, except as noted:
chum or coho *(Peter Pan)* 90
king *(Peter Pan)* 140
Norwegian fillet *(Abelvaer)*, 3 oz. 170
pink, skinless fillet *(Chicken of the Sea)*, 2 oz. 60
red *(Peter Pan)* 110
red, blueback *(Rubinstein's)* 110
red, sockeye *(S&W)*, 3¾-oz. can 190
Salmon, frozen:
chum, fillet or steak *(Peter Pan)*, 4 oz. 130
coho, fillet *(Peter Pan)*, 4 oz. 160
Salmon, smoked:
chinook, lox, 4 oz. 133
lox, Nova, natural or w/color *(Vita)*, 2 oz. 50
Salmon, smoked, spread *(Vita)*, ¼ cup, 2 oz. 180
Salsa, 2 tbsp., except as noted:
(Marie's Tomato) 10

all varieties *(Del Monte)* 10
all varieties *(Old El Paso* Regular) 10
all varieties *(Old El Paso* Thick 'n Chunky) 15
all varieties *(Pace)* 10
all varieties *(Rosarita/Rosarita* Extra Chunky/Traditional) . . 10
all varieties *(S&W* Ready-Cut), ¼ cup 20
con queso *(Tostitos/Tostitos* Low Fat) 40
garlic, roasted *(Marie's)* 10
garlic, roasted *(Tostitos)* 15
mild, medium and ultimate *(Tostitos)* 15
picante (see also "Picante sauce") *(Old Dutch)* 10
sweet and zesty *(Tostitos)* 20
Salsa, fruit, see specific fruit listings
Salsa seasoning *(Lawry's)*, ½ tsp. 5
Salsify:
raw *(Frieda's)*, ¾ cup, 3 oz. 70
boiled, drained, sliced, ½ cup 46
Salt, iodized or noniodized *(Morton)*, ¼ tsp. 0
Salt pork, raw, 1 oz. 212
Sandwich sauce, ¼ cup:
(Manwich Original) 30
(Manwich Barbecue/Bold) 60
(Manwich Thick & Chunky) 45
Mexican *(Manwich)* 25
Sloppy joe *(Del Monte* Original/Hickory) 70
Sloppy joe *(Green Giant)* 50
Sloppy joe, and meat *(Green Giant)* 200
Sandwich spread *(Kraft* Spread & Burger Sauce),
  1 tbsp. 50
Sapodilla, 1 medium, 3 ∞2½ 140
Sapote, 1 medium, 11.2 oz. 301
Sardine, fresh, see "Herring"
Sardine, canned:
in mustard sauce *(Underwood)*, 3¾-oz. can 180
in olive oil, drained:
    Norway brisling *(S&W)*, 3¾-oz. can 160
    skinless, boneless *(Granadaisa)*, ¼ cup 120
    skinless, boneless *(S&W)*, 3¾-oz. can 100
in soy oil, drained *(Underwood)*, 3 oz. 220
spiced or in lemon *(Goya)*, ¼ cup 120

Sardine, canned *(cont.)*

in tomato sauce *(Del Monte),* 2 oz., ½ fish w/sauce 80

in tomato sauce *(Underwood),* 3¾ oz. 180

Sauce, see specific listings

Sauerkraut, w/liquid, ½ cup 22

Sauerkraut juice *(S&W),* 10-oz. can 35

Sausage (see also specific listings), cooked:

beef, smoked *(Oscar Mayer* Smokies), 1 link 120

brown and serve *(Little Sizzlers),* 3 links 230

brown and serve *(Little Sizzlers),* 2 patties 190

cheese, smoked *(Oscar Mayer* Little Smokies), 6 links . 180

dinner *(Jones Dairy Farm),* 1 link 210

dinner *(Jones Dairy Farm* All Natural), 1 link 130

dinner, Italian *(Jones Dairy Farm),* 1 link 140

Italian style, pork, hot *(Garden State),* 1 link 160

Italian style, hot, crumbles *(Johnsville),* 2 oz. 170

Italian style, sweet *(Garden State),* 1 link 180

Mexican style, pork, crumbles *(Johnsville),* 2 oz. 160

pickled, smoked or hot *(Hormel),* 6 links 140

pork links (see also specific sausage listings):

    (Little Sizzlers), 3 links 180

    (Oscar Mayer), 2 links 180

    breakfast *(Garden State),* 3 links 300

    breakfast, apple cinnamon, or Vermont maple syrup

       (Johnsville), 3 links 200

    hot and spicy *(Little Sizzlers),* 3 links 180

pork patties *(Little Sizzlers),* 2 patties 210

pork roll *(Jones Dairy Farm* All Natural), 2 oz. 230

smoked *(Boar's Head),* 4.5 oz. 400

smoked *(John Morrell* Bun Size), 1 link 270

smoked *(John Morrell* Bun Size Less Fat), 1 link 180

smoked *(Oscar Mayer* Little Smokies), 6 links 170

smoked, hot *(Boar's Head),* 3.2 oz. 280

"Sausage," vegetarian:

canned *(Loma Linda* Little Links), 2 links 90

canned *(Worthington Saucettes),* 1 link 90

frozen:

    (Morningstar Farms Breakfast), 2 links 60

    (Morningstar Farms Breakfast), 1 patty 70

    (Worthington Prosage Links), 2 links 60

(Worthington Prosage Patties), 1 patty 100
crumbles *(Morningstar Farms* Recipe Crumbles),
　2/3 cup 90
crumbles *(Natural Touch* Vegan Crumbles), 1/2 cup . . 60
roll *(Worthington Prosage)*, 5/8 slice 140
Sausage hash, canned *(Mary Kitchen),* 1 cup 410
Sausage stick, 1 piece, except as noted:
beef *(Boar's Head),* .6 oz. 100
beef *(Rustlers Roundup* Jerky), .2 oz. 30
beef or summer *(Old Dutch),* 1 oz. 110
hot *(Rustlers Roundup),* .3 oz. 40
smoked *(Rustlers Roundup* Steak Stick), .8 oz. 60
smoked, mild or spicy *(Slim Jim),* 1.4-oz. box 210
spicy *(Rustlers Roundup),* .5 oz. 50
Savory, ground *(McCormick),* 1/4 tsp. 2
Scallion, see "Onion, green"
Scallop, meat only:
raw, 2 large or 5 small, 1.1 oz. 26
frozen *(Tyson* Delight), 1/2 cup 80
Scallop, fried, frozen *(Mrs. Paul's),* 12 pieces 200
"Scallop," vegetarian, canned:
(Loma Linda Tender Bits), 6 pieces 110
(Worthington Vegetable Skallops), 1/2 cup 90
Scallop squash, boiled, drained, sliced, 1/2 cup 14
Scone, all varieties *(Health Valley),* 1 piece 180
Scrapple *(Jones Dairy Farm),* 2 oz. 120
Scrod, fresh, see "Cod, Atlantic"
Scup, meat only, baked or broiled, 4 oz. 153
Sea bass, meat only, baked or broiled, 4 oz. 141
Sea trout, meat only, baked or broiled, 4 oz. 151
Seafood cocktail sauce, 1/4 cup, except as noted:
(Bookbinder's Restaurant Style/Hot and Spicy) 70
(Heinz) 60
(Heluva Good) 40
(Maull's), 2 tbsp. 45
(S&W), 1 tsp. 20
Seasoning and coating mix, see specific listings
Seaweed:
agar, flakes or bar *(Eden),* 1 tbsp. 10
arame or hiziki *(Eden),* 1/2 cup 30

Seaweed *(cont.)*
kombu *(Eden)*, ½ of 7˝ piece 10
nori *(Eden)*, 1 sheet 10
wakame *(Eden)*, ½ cup 25
Semolina flour, mix *(Arrowhead Mills)*, ½ cup 240
Sesame meal, partially defatted, 1 oz. 161
Sesame paste, see "Tahini"
Sesame seasoning, all varieties *(Eden)*, ½ tsp. 10
Sesame seeds, ¼ cup:
whole, brown *(Arrowhead Mills)* 200
kernels *(Arrowhead Mills)* 210
Shad, meat only, baked or broiled, 4 oz. 286
Shallot:
fresh, peeled *(Frieda's)*, 1 tbsp., 1.1 oz. 20
freeze-dried *(McCormick)*, ¼ tsp. 3
Shark, meat only, raw, 4 oz. 148
Sheepshead, meat only, baked or broiled, 4 oz. 143
Shellie beans, canned *(Stokely)*, ½ cup 45
Shells, pasta:
refrigerated *(Tutta Pasta)*, ⅞ cup 300
and cheese *(Stouffer)*, ½ of 12-oz. pkg. 260
Shells, pasta, entree, frozen, marinara *(Healthy
Choice)*, 12 oz. 390
Shells, pasta, mix, approx. 1 cup*:
and cheese *(Velveeta Original/With Bacon)* 360
and cheese, w/salsa *(Velveeta Original)* 380
creamy, and cheese *(Land O Lakes Dinner)* 350
white cheddar *(Pasta Roni)* 390
Sherbet (see also "Ice" and "Sorbet"), ½ cup:
pink lemonade *(Dreyer's)* 120
strawberry kiwi *(Edy's/Dreyer's)* 120
Swiss orange or raz chip *(Edy's/Dreyer's)* 150
tangerine *(Edy's)* 130
tropical *(Edy's/Dreyer's)* 130
Sherbet cup, orange *(Sealtest)*, 4-oz. cup 130
Sherbet smoothie, 1 piece:
strawberry fields *(Dreyer's)* 90
tropical oasis *(Dreyer's)* 100
Shortening *(Pillsbury/Snowdrift/Swiftening)*, 1 tbsp. . . . 110

Shrimp, meat only:
raw, 4 large, 1 oz. 30
boiled or steamed, 4 oz. 112
boiled or steamed, 4 large 22
Shrimp, canned, small or medium *(S&W),* ¼ cup 45
"Shrimp," imitation, frozen, jumbo *(Captain Jac*
   Shrimp Tasties), 3 pieces, 3 oz. 90
Shrimp cocktail *(Sau-Sea),* 6-oz. jar 150
Shrimp dinner, frozen:
marinara *(Healthy Choice),* 10.5 oz. 250
Mariner *(The Budget Gourmet),* 11 oz. 270
and vegetables Maria *(Healthy Choice),* 12.5 oz. 290
Shrimp entree, canned *(La Choy* Chow Mein), 1 cup . . .50
Shrimp entree, frozen:
batter, beer *(Gorton's),* 6 pieces 250
breaded *(Gorton's),* 6 pieces 230
breaded *(Mrs. Paul's),* 1 pkg. 350
breaded *(Van de Kamp's),* 7 pieces, 4 oz. 240
breaded, butterfly *(Van de Kamp's),* 7 pieces 280
breaded, scampi *(Gorton's),* 6 pieces 250
marinara *(Smart Ones),* 9 oz. 190
popcorn *(Gorton's),* 1 cup, 3.2 oz. 260
popcorn *(Gorton's),* 1¼ cups, 3.5 oz. 270
popcorn *(Van de Kamp's),* 20 pieces, 4 oz. 270
Sloppy joe sauce, see "Sandwich sauce"
Smelt, rainbow, meat only, baked or broiled, 4 oz. 141
Snack mix:
(Cheez-It), ½ cup 140
(Chex Mix), ⅔ cup 130
(Chex Mix Bold n' Zesty), ½ cup 150
(Old Dutch Party Mix), ⅔ cup 150
(Pepperidge Farm Light Season), ½ cup 170
cheddar *(Chex Mix),* ⅔ cup 140
Snail, sea, see "Whelk"
Snapper, meat only, baked or broiled, 4 oz. 145
Snow pea, see "Peas, edible-podded"
Sofrito, see "Soup base"
Soft drinks, carbonated, 12 fl. oz., except as noted:
all varieties *(R.W. Knudsen Fruit TeaZer)* 110
all varieties, sparkling *(Santa Cruz)* 150

Soft drinks *(cont.)*

apple, boysenberry, or lime *(R.W. Knudsen* Spritzer) . . . 160
apple, spiced *(Natural Brew)* 170
birch beer *(Canada Dry)*, 8 fl. oz. 110
cafe mocha *(Natural Brew)* 150
*(Canada Dry Hi-Spot/*Cactus Cooler), 8 fl. oz. 110
cherry *(Sundrop)* 180
cherry, black *(After the Fall* Spritzer) 170
cherry, black *(Canada Dry)*, 8 fl. oz. 130
cherry, black *(Shasta)* 170
cherry, French *(Snapple)*, 8 fl. oz. 120
cherry, wild *(Canada Dry)*, 8 fl. oz. 110
cherry spice *(Slice)* 150
cherry-lime *(Spree)* 170
cherry-lime rickey *(Snapple)*, 8 fl. oz. 110
chocolate, noncarbonated, see "Chocolate drink"
citrus *(Canada Dry* Half & Half), 8 fl. oz. 110
club soda or seltzer 0
cola *(Pepsi/Pepsi* Caffeine Free) 150
cola *(Shasta)* 170
cola, cherry *(R.W. Knudsen* Spritzer) 170
cola, cherry *(Shasta)* 160
cola, cherry, wild *(Pepsi)* 160
cola, ginseng *(Natural Brew)* 170
collins mixer *(Schweppes)*, 8 fl. oz. 100
cranberry *(R.W. Knudsen* Spritzer) 190
cranberry *(Shasta)* 180
cream *(A&W)*, 8 fl. oz. 110
cream *(Hires)* 180
cream, vanilla *(Canada Dry)*, 8 fl. oz. 120
cream, vanilla *(Snapple* Creme D'Vanilla), 8 fl. oz. 130
(Doc Shasta) 160
(Dr Pepper) 160
fruit punch *(Canada Dry* Tahitian), 8 fl. oz. 150
fruit punch *(Juice Fizz)*, 8 fl. oz. 130
fruit punch *(Shasta)* 200
fruit punch, tropical *(Spree)* 170
ginger ale *(Canada Dry/Schweppes)*, 8 fl. oz. 90
ginger ale *(Canada Dry* Cherry/Golden), 8 fl. oz. 100
ginger ale *(Natural Brew* Outrageous) 170

ginger ale *(Shasta)* 130
ginger ale, grape or raspberry *(Schweppes)*, 8 fl. oz. . . . 100
ginger beer *(Goya)* 190
grape *(Canada Dry* Concord), 8 fl. oz. 120
grape *(R.W. Knudsen* Spritzer) 170
grape *(Shasta)* 190
grapefruit *(Shasta* Ruby Red) 190
grapefruit *(Spree)* 170
kiwi-lime *(R.W. Knudsen* Spritzer) 160
lemon, bitter or sour *(Schweppes)*, 8 fl. oz. 110
lemon, sour *(Canada Dry)*, 8 fl. oz. 100
lemonade or lemon-lime *(R.W. Knudsen* Spritzer) 170
lemon-lime *(Schweppes)*, 8 fl. oz. 100
lemon-lime *(Slice)* 150
lime-lemon *(Shasta Twist)* 150
mango *(R.W. Knudsen* Fandango Spritzer) 190
mango ginger *(After the Fall* Spritzer) 150
(Mountain Dew/Mountain Dew Caffeine Free) 170
orange *(Canada Dry* Sunripe), 8 fl. oz. 140
orange *(Crush)* 200
orange *(Orangina)*, 10 fl. oz. 120
orange *(Shasta)* 200
orange creme *(Natural Brews)* 160
orange–passion fruit or peach *(R.W. Knudsen* Spritzer) . 160
peach *(Shasta)* 170
peach *(Snapple* Melba), 8 fl. oz. 120
peach vanilla *(After the Fall* Spritzer) 170
pineapple *(Canada Dry)*, 8 fl. oz. 110
pineapple *(Shasta)* 200
pineapple *(Sunkist)*, 8 fl. oz. 140
pineapple-orange *(Shasta)* 180
raspberry *(After the Fall* Spritzer) 170
red or raspberry creme *(Shasta)* 170
root beer *(A&W)*, 8 fl. oz. 110
root beer *(Hires)* 180
root beer *(Mug)* 160
root beer *(Snapple* Tru), 8 fl. oz. 110
(7Up/7Up Cherry) 160
sour mixer *(Canada Dry)*, 8 fl. oz. 90
strawberry *(Canada Dry* California), 8 fl. oz. 110

Soft drinks *(cont.)*
strawberry *(R.W. Knudsen* Spritzer) 170
strawberry *(Sunkist),* 8 fl. oz. 140
strawberry peach *(Shasta)* 170
strawberry vanilla *(After the Fall* Spritzer) 160
(Sundrop) 200
tangerine spritzer *(After the Fall/R.W. Knudsen)* 170
tonic *(Shasta)* 170
tonic, plain or flavored *(Schweppes),* 8 fl. oz. 90
vanilla bean *(After the Fall* Spritzer) 170
Sole:
fresh, baked, broiled, or microwaved, 4 oz. 133
frozen *(Van de Kamp's* Natural), 4-oz. fillet 110
Sole entree, breaded, frozen:
(Mrs. Paul's Premium), 1 fillet 250
(Van de Kamp's Light), 1 fillet 220
Sopressata *(Boar's Head Cinghiale* Mini), 1 oz. 100
Sorbet (see also "Ice" and "Sherbet"), ½ cup:
all flavors *(Colombo)* 100
banana strawberry *(Häagen-Dazs)* 140
cherry *(Sharon's Sorbet)* 95
cherry cordial *(Edy's/Dreyer's* Whole Fruit) 160
chocolate *(Häagen-Dazs)* 130
chocolate *(Tofutti)* 90
chocolate, Dutch *(Sharon's Sorbet)* 90
coconut *(Sharon's Sorbet)* 100
coffee *(Sharon's Sorbet)* 100
coffee *(Tofutti)* 80
cranberry-orange *(Ben & Jerry's)* 130
and cream, orange or raspberry *(Häagen-Dazs)* 190
devil's food *(Ben & Jerry's)* 160
lemon *(Edy's/Dreyer's* Whole Fruit) 140
lemon *(Häagen-Dazs Zesty Lemon)* 120
lemon *(Sharon's Sorbet)* 75
mango or raspberry *(Häagen-Dazs)* 120
mango-lime *(Ben & Jerry's)* 130
mango-orange *(Edy's/Dreyer's* Whole Fruit) 120
orange-peach-mango *(Tofutti)* 90
passion fruit *(Sharon's Sorbet)* 80
peach *(Edy's/Dreyer's* Whole Fruit) 130

peach *(Häagen-Dazs Orchard)* 140
peach *(Sharon's Sorbet)* 75
piña colada *(Ben & Jerry's)* 140
purple passion *(Ben & Jerry's)* 120
raspberry *(Edy's/Dreyer's Whole Fruit)* 130
raspberry *(Sharon's Sorbet)* 80
strawberry *(Edy's/Dreyer's Whole Fruit)* 120
strawberry *(Häagen-Dazs)* 130
strawberry *(Tofutti)* 80
strawberry kiwi *(Ben & Jerry's)* 130
Sorbet bar, 1 bar:
berry, wild *(Häagen-Dazs)* 90
chocolate *(Häagen-Dazs)* 80
Sorbet and yogurt bar, 1 bar:
banana-strawberry or raspberry-vanilla *(Häagen-Dazs)* . 90
chocolate-cherry *(Häagen-Dazs)* 100
Soup, canned, ready-to-serve, 1 cup, except as noted:
bean *(Grandma Brown's)* 190
bean, black *(Health Valley/Health Valley Organic)* 110
bean, black, hearty *(Progresso)* 170
bean, salsa *(Campbell's Home Cookin')* 160
bean and ham *(Campbell's Home Cookin')* 180
bean and ham *(Healthy Choice)* 160
bean and ham *(Progresso)* 160
bean and ham, hearty *(Campbell's Chunky)* 190
bean vegetable, 5 *(Health Valley)* 140
beef, pasta *(Campbell's Chunky)* 150
beef, potato *(Healthy Choice)* 110
beef barley *(Progresso)* 130
beef barley *(Progresso 99% Fat Free)* 140
beef broth *(College Inn)* 20
beef broth *(Swanson)* 20
beef minestrone or noodle *(Progresso)* 140
beef vegetable *(Progresso 99% Fat Free)* 160
beef vegetable and rotini *(Progresso)* 130
beef w/vegetables, country *(Campbell's Chunky)* 160
broccoli cheese *(Healthy Choice)* 110
broccoli and shells *(Progresso Pasta Soup)* 80
chicken *(Progresso Chickarina)* 120
chicken Alfredo *(Healthy Choice)* 120

Soup, canned, ready-to-serve *(cont.)*

chicken, cream of, w/vegetables *(Healthy Choice)* 120
chicken, hearty *(Healthy Choice)* 130
chicken barley, minestrone, or vegetable *(Progresso)* . . . 100
chicken broccoli cheese *(Campbell's Chunky)* 200
chicken broth *(Campbell's Healthy Request)* 20
chicken broth *(College Inn/College Inn Less Sodium)* 25
chicken broth *(Swanson)* 30
chicken broth *(Swanson Natural Goodness)* 15
chicken corn chowder *(Campbell's Chunky)* 250
chicken corn chowder *(Healthy Choice)* 160
chicken mushroom chowder *(Campbell's Chunky)* 210
chicken noodle *(Campbell's Chunky Classic)* 130
chicken noodle *(Campbell's Glass Jar)* 80
chicken noodle *(Healthy Choice)* 150
chicken noodle *(Progresso)* 80
chicken noodle *(Progresso 99% Fat Free)* 90
chicken noodle, egg noodle *(Campbell's Home Cookin')* . . 90
chicken noodle, hearty *(Campbell's Healthy Request)* . . . 100
chicken pasta *(Campbell's Glass Jar)* 90
chicken pasta *(Healthy Choice)* 120
chicken pasta, w/mushroom *(Campbell's Chunky)* 120
chicken and penne, spicy *(Progresso Pasta Soup)* 110
chicken rice *(Campbell's Home Cookin')* 110
chicken rice *(Healthy Choice)* 100
chicken rice, hearty *(Campbell's Healthy Request)* 110
chicken rice, savory *(Campbell's Chunky)* 140
chicken rice, w/vegetables *(Progresso)* 100
chicken rice, w/vegetables *(Progresso 99% Fat Free)* 90
chicken and rotini *(Progresso Pasta Soup)* 90
chicken vegetable *(Campbell's Home Cookin')* 130
chicken vegetable, hearty *(Campbell's Healthy Request)* . 110
chicken vegetable, spicy *(Campbell's Chunky)* 90
chicken w/vegetables, hearty *(Campbell's Chunky)* 90
chicken w/vegetables, homestyle *(Progresso)* 80
chicken and wild rice *(Progresso)* 90
chili beef *(Healthy Choice)* 170
chili beef w/beans *(Campbell's Chunky)*, 11 oz. 300
clam chowder:
    Manhattan *(Progresso)* 110

New England *(Campbell's* Chunky) 240
New England *(Campbell's* Home Cookin') 200
New England *(Campbell's Healthy Request)* 120
New England *(Healthy Choice)* 120
New England *(Progresso)* 200
New England *(Progresso* 99% Fat Free) 130
clam and rotini chowder *(Progresso* Pasta Soup) 190
corn, country, and vegetable *(Health Valley)* 70
escarole, in chicken broth *(Progresso)* 25
gumbo, zesty *(Healthy Choice)* 100
hot and sour *(Rice Road)* 90
lentil *(Health Valley* Organic) 90
lentil *(Healthy Choice)* 140
lentil *(Progresso)* 140
lentil *(Progresso* 99% Fat Free) 130
lentil, savory *(Campbell's* Home Cookin') 130
lentil and shells *(Progresso* Pasta Soup) 130
macaroni and bean *(Progresso)* 160
meatballs and pasta pearls *(Progresso)* 140
minestrone *(Campbell's* Chunky/Home Cookin') 140
minestrone *(Campbell's* Glass Jar) 120
minestrone *(Healthy Choice)* 110
minestrone *(Progresso)* 120
minestrone *(Progresso* 99% Fat Free) 130
minestrone, hearty *(Campbell's Healthy Request)* 120
minestrone, Parmesan *(Progresso)* 100
minestrone, Tuscany *(Campbell's* Home Cookin') 160
mushroom, cream of *(Campbell's* Glass Jar) 260
mushroom, cream of *(Healthy Choice)* 80
mushroom barley *(Health Valley* Organic) 60
mushroom chicken, creamy *(Progresso* 99% Fat Free) . . 90
mushroom and rice *(Campbell's* Home Cookin') 80
pasta, Bolognese or cacciatore *(Health Valley Healthy
   Pasta)* 100
pasta, fagioli *(Health Valley Healthy Pasta)* 120
pasta, primavera *(Health Valley Healthy Pasta)* 110
pasta, Romano or rotini-vegetable *(Health Valley
   Healthy Pasta)* 100
pea, split *(Grandma Brown's)* 210
pea, split, or green split *(Progresso)* 170

Soup, canned, ready-to-serve *(cont.)*
pea, split, and carrots *(Health Valley)* 110
pea, split, w/ham *(Campbell's Chunky)* 190
pea, split, w/ham *(Campbell's Healthy Request/Home
   Cookin')* 170
pea, split, w/ham *(Healthy Choice)* 160
pea, split, w/ham *(Progresso)* 150
penne, hearty, in chicken broth *(Progresso Pasta Soup)* . . 90
penne, zesty *(Campbell's Healthy Request)* 90
pepper steak *(Campbell's Chunky)* 140
potato, baked *(Healthy Choice)* 140
potato, w/roasted garlic *(Campbell's Home Cookin')* 180
potato ham chowder *(Campbell's Chunky)* 220
potato leek *(Health Valley Organic)* 70
sirloin burger, w/vegetable *(Campbell's Chunky)* 180
steak and potato *(Campbell's Chunky)* 160
tomato, garden *(Healthy Choice)* 100
tomato, hearty, and rotini *(Progresso Pasta Soup)* 130
tomato, tortellini *(Progresso Pasta Soup)* 120
tomato vegetable *(Progresso)* 90
tomato vegetable, garden *(Progresso 99% Fat Free)* . . . 100
tomato vegetable, w/pasta *(Campbell's Healthy
   Request)* 120
tortellini, in chicken broth *(Progresso)* 70
tortellini, w/chicken and vegetables *(Campbell's
   Chunky)* 110
turkey vegetable w/wild rice *(Campbell's Healthy
   Request)* 120
turkey w/white and wild rice *(Healthy Choice)* 90
vegetable *(Campbell's Chunky)* 130
vegetable *(Progresso)* 90
vegetable *(Progresso 99% Fat Free)* 80
vegetable, country *(Campbell's Home Cookin')* 110
vegetable, country *(Healthy Choice)* 100
vegetable, garden *(Healthy Choice)* 120
vegetable, 14 garden *(Health Valley Fat Free)* 80
vegetable, harborside *(Campbell's Home Cookin')* 80
vegetable, hearty *(Campbell's Healthy Request)* 100
vegetable, hearty, w/pasta *(Campbell's Chunky)* 140
vegetable, hearty, and rotini *(Progresso Pasta Soup)* . . . 110

vegetable, Italian *(Campbell's* Home Cookin') 100
vegetable, Southwest, w/black beans *(Campbell's*
   Healthy Request) 140
vegetable, vegetarian *(Pritikin)* 100
vegetable barley *(Health Valley* Fat Free) 90
vegetable beef *(Campbell's* Chunky) 150
vegetable beef *(Campbell's* Home Cookin') 120
vegetable beef *(Healthy Choice)* 120
vegetable beef, hearty *(Campbell's Healthy Request)* . . . 140
vegetable beef, w/pasta *(Campbell's* Glass Jar) 110
vegetable broth *(College Inn)* 20
vegetable broth *(Swanson)* 20
vegetable and pasta *(Campbell's* Glass Jar) 110
Soup, canned, condensed, undiluted, ½ cup:
asparagus, cream of *(Campbell's)* 90
bean, w/bacon *(Campbell's)* 180
bean, w/bacon *(Campbell's Healthy Request)* 150
bean, black *(Campbell's)* 120
beef, w/vegetables and barley *(Campbell's)* 80
beef broth, double rich *(Campbell's)* 15
beef consommé *(Campbell's)* 25
beef noodle *(Campbell's)* 70
broccoli, cream of *(Campbell's)* 100
broccoli, cream of *(Campbell's Healthy Request)* 70
broccoli, cream of/cheese *(Campbell's* 98% Fat Free) . . . 80
broccoli cheddar *(Campbell's Healthy Request Creative*
   Chef) 80
broccoli cheddar *(Healthy Choice)* 90
broccoli cheese *(Campbell's)* 110
celery, cream of *(Campbell's)* 110
celery, cream of *(Campbell's* 98% Fat Free/*Healthy*
   Request) 70
celery, cream of *(Healthy Choice)* 70
cheese, cheddar *(Campbell's)* 90
cheese, nacho *(Campbell's)* 140
chicken, cream of:
   (Campbell's) 130
   (Campbell's 98% Fat Free) 80
   (Campbell's Healthy Request/Creative Chef) 80
   and broccoli *(Campbell's)* 120

Soup, canned, condensed, chicken, cream of *(cont.)*

and broccoli *(Campbell's Healthy Request)* 80
roasted *(Healthy Choice)* 90
roasted, w/herbs *(Campbell's Healthy Request
  Creative Chef)* 80
chicken alphabet, w/vegetables *(Campbell's)* 80
chicken broth *(Campbell's)* 30
chicken dumplings *(Campbell's)* 80
chicken gumbo *(Campbell's)* 60
chicken mushroom, creamy *(Campbell's)* 130
chicken noodle *(Campbell's/Campbell's Healthy
  Request)* 70
chicken noodle, creamy *(Campbell's)* 130
chicken noodle, curly/O's *(Campbell's)* 80
chicken noodle, homestyle *(Campbell's)* 70
chicken w/rice or white/wild rice *(Campbell's)* 70
chicken w/rice *(Campbell's Healthy Request)* 60
chicken and stars *(Campbell's)* 70
chicken vegetable *(Campbell's/Campbell's Healthy
  Request)* 80
chicken vegetable, Southwestern *(Campbell's)* 110
chili beef and bean *(Campbell's)* 170
clam chowder, Manhattan *(Bookbinder's)* 80
clam chowder, Manhattan *(Campbell's)* 60
clam chowder, New England *(Campbell's/Campbell's
  98% Fat Free)* 90
clam chowder, New England *(Doxsee)* 90
corn, golden *(Campbell's)* 120
crab bisque *(Bookbinder's)* 120
garlic, roasted, cream of *(Healthy Choice)* 60
lobster bisque *(Bookbinder's)* 90
minestrone *(Campbell's/Campbell's Healthy Request)* . . . 90
mushroom, beefy *(Campbell's)* 70
mushroom, cream of *(Campbell's)* 110
mushroom, cream of *(Campbell's 98% Fat Free/
  Campbell's Healthy Request/Healthy Request
  Creative Chef)* 70
mushroom, cream of *(Healthy Choice)* 60
mushroom, golden *(Campbell's)* 80
noodle, double, chicken broth *(Campbell's)* 100

noodles and ground beef *(Campbell's)* 100
onion, cream of *(Campbell's)* 110
onion, French, w/beef stock *(Campbell's)* 70
oyster stew *(Bookbinder's)* 90
oyster stew *(Campbell's)* 90
pea, green or split w/ham *(Campbell's)* 180
pepper, cream of Mexican *(Campbell's)* 110
pepperpot *(Campbell's)* 100
potato, cream of *(Campbell's)* 90
potato, cream of herbed, w/roasted garlic *(Campbell's*
   Healthy Request Creative Chef) 80
Scotch broth *(Campbell's)* 80
seafood bisque *(Bookbinder's)* 140
shrimp, cream of *(Campbell's)* 100
shrimp bisque *(Bookbinder's)* 120
snapper *(Bookbinder's)* 110
tomato *(Campbell's)* 80
tomato *(Campbell's Healthy Request)* 90
tomato *(Healthy Choice)* 80
tomato, fiesta *(Campbell's)* 70
tomato, w/garden herbs *(Campbell's Healthy Request*
   Creative Chef) 100
tomato, Italian, w/basil, oregano *(Campbell's)* 100
tomato bisque *(Campbell's)* 130
tomato rice *(Campbell's* Old Fashioned) 120
turkey, noodle or vegetable *(Campbell's)* 80
vegetable *(Campbell's/Campbell's Healthy Request)* . . . 90
vegetable *(Campbell's* Old Fashioned) 70
vegetable, California style *(Campbell's)* 60
vegetable, hearty, w/pasta *(Campbell's/Campbell's*
   Healthy Request) 90
vegetable, vegetarian *(Campbell's)* 60
vegetable beef *(Campbell's/Campbell's Healthy Request)* . . 80
wonton *(Campbell's)* 45
Soup, mix, dry, 1 pkg., except as noted:
barley, better *(Aunt Patsy's Pantry)*, 2 tbsp. 90
bean, black *(Aunt Patsy's Pantry)*, 1/6 pkg. 190
bean, black *(Bean Cuisine* Island), 1 serving 126
bean, black, spicy, w/couscous *(Health Valley)*, 1/3 cup . 130
bean, black, zesty, w/rice *(Health Valley)*, 1/3 cup 100

Soup, mix *(cont.)*
bean, 5, hearty *(Fantastic Foods)*, 2.3 oz. 230
bean and ham *(Hormel Micro Cup)* 190
beef vegetable *(Hormel Micro Cup)* 90
broccoli-cheese, creamy *(Cup-a-Soup)* 70
broccoli-cheese, w/ham *(Hormel Micro Cup)* 170
chicken, cream of *(Cup-a-Soup)* 70
chicken broth *(Cup-a-Soup)* 20
chicken broth, w/pasta *(Cup-a-Soup)* 45
chicken noodle:
    (Campbell's Real Chicken Broth), 3 tbsp. 100
    (Campbell's Soup and Recipe), 3 tbsp. 90
    (Cup-a-Soup) 50
    (Hormel Micro Cup) 110
    double *(Campbell's)* 170
    hearty *(Cup-a-Soup)* 60
chicken onion *(Lipton Soup Secrets Kettle Style)*,
    1 cup* 120
chicken rice *(Hormel Micro Cup)* 110
chicken rice *(Mrs. Grass)*, ¼ pkg. 80
chili *(Aunt Patsy's Pantry Cowgirl)*, 4 tbsp. 160
chili, black bean *(Aunt Patsy's Pantry)*, 3 tbsp. 100
chili, chicken *(Aunt Patsy's Pantry)*, 4 tbsp. 180
clam chowder, New England *(Hormel Micro Cup)* 130
corn chowder *(Smart Soup)* 100
corn chowder, w/tomatoes *(Health Valley)*, ½ cup 90
couscous *(Casbah Moroccan Stew Cup)* 180
couscous, black bean salsa *(Fantastic)*, 2.4 oz. 240
couscous, cheddar, nacho *(Fantastic)*, 1.9 oz. 200
couscous, corn, sweet *(Fantastic)*, 1.8 oz. 180
couscous, vegetable, Creole *(Fantastic)*, 2.1 oz. 220
herb, 1 cup*:
    fiesta, w/red pepper *(Lipton Recipe Secrets)* 30
    w/garlic, savory *(Lipton Recipe Secrets)* 30
    golden, w/lemon *(Lipton Recipe Secrets)* 35
    Italian, w/tomato *(Lipton Recipe Secrets)* 40
lentil *(Smart Soup)* 190
lentil, homestyle *(Lipton Soup Secrets Kettle Style)*,
    1 cup* 130
lentil, red *(Aunt Patsy's Pantry)*, 2 tbsp. 80

lentil, w/couscous *(Health Valley)*, ⅓ cup 130
minestrone *(Lipton Soup Secrets* Kettle Style), 1 cup* . 110
minestrone *(Smart Soup)* 120
minestrone, hearty *(Fantastic)*, 1.5 oz. 150
mushroom, beefy *(Lipton Recipe Secrets)*, 1½ tbsp. 35
mushroom, creamy *(Cup-a-Soup)* 60
mushroom, creamy *(Fantastic)*, 1.2 oz. 120
noodle *(Nissin Top Ramen* Damae/Oriental) 190
noodle, beef *(Nissin Cup Noodles)* 300
noodle, beef *(Nissin Top Ramen)* 190
noodle, beef, picante *(Nissin Top Ramen)* 180
noodle, chicken *(Lipton Soup Secrets)*, 2 tbsp. 60
noodle, chicken *(Lipton Soup Secrets* Giggle/
   Ring-O-Noodle), 1 cup* 70
noodle, chicken *(Nissin Cup Noodles)* 300
noodle, chicken *(Nissin Top Ramen)* 180
noodle, chicken broth *(Lipton Soup Secrets)*, 2 tbsp. . . . 60
noodle, chicken broth *(Mrs. Grass)*, ¼ pkg. 60
noodle, w/chicken broth *(Mrs. Grass)*, ¼ pkg. 60
noodle, chicken, Cajun *(Nissin Cup Noodles)* 300
noodle, chicken, Cajun *(Nissin Top Ramen)* 180
noodle, chicken, creamy *(Nissin Cup Noodles)* 300
noodle, chicken, creamy *(Nissin Top Ramen)* 190
noodle, chicken, mushroom *(Nissin Cup Noodles)* 300
noodle, chicken, mushroom *(Nissin Top Ramen)* 190
noodle, chicken, sesame *(Nissin Top Ramen)* 190
noodle, chicken, spicy *(Nissin Cup Noodles)* 300
noodle, chicken, w/vegetables *(Health Valley)*, ⅓ cup . . . 80
noodle, chicken free *(Fantastic)*, 1.5 oz. 140
noodle, w/chicken meat *(Lipton Soup Secrets)*, 1 cup* . . 80
noodle, chicken teriyaki *(Nissin Cup Noodles)* 300
noodle, chicken teriyaki *(Nissin Top Ramen)* 190
noodle, chicken vegetable *(Nissin Cup Noodles)* 300
noodle, chicken vegetable *(Nissin Top Ramen)* 190
noodle, extra *(Lipton Soup Secrets)*, 1 cup* 90
noodle, French onion *(Nissin Cup Noodles)* 300
noodle, Oriental *(Campbell's/Sanwa* Ramen), ½ block . 170
noodle, pork *(Campbell's* Ramen), ½ block 170
noodle, ring noodle *(Cup-a-Soup)* 50
noodle, seafood *(Nissin Cup Noodles)* 300

Soup, mix *(cont.)*

noodle, shrimp *(Nissin Cup Noodles)* 300
noodle, shrimp *(Nissin Top Ramen)* 190
noodle, shrimp, picante *(Nissin Cup Noodles)* 310
noodle, smoked ham *(Nissin Cup Noodles)* 300
noodle, smoked ham *(Nissin Top Ramen)* 180
noodle, vegetable, tomato *(Fantastic)*, 1.5 oz. 150
noodle, vegetable beef *(Mrs. Grass)*, ¼ pkg. 70
onion *(Campbell's Soup and Recipe)*, 1 tbsp. 20
onion *(Lipton Recipe Secrets)*, 1 cup* 20
onion *(Mrs. Grass Soup/Recipe)*, ¼ pkg. 35
onion, beefy *(Lipton Recipe Secrets)*, 1 cup* 25
onion, golden *(Lipton Recipe Secrets)*, 1⅔ tbsp. 50
onion-mushroom *(Lipton Recipe Secrets)*, 1 cup* 30
onion-mushroom *(Mrs. Grass Soup/Recipe)*, ¼ pkg. . . . 60
pasta, Italiano *(Health Valley* Fat Free*)*, ½ cup 140
pasta, marinara, Mediterranean, or Parmesan *(Health
   Valley* Pasta Cup Fat Free*)*, ½ cup 100
pasta, spiral *(Lipton Soup Secrets)*, 3 tbsp. 60
pasta and white bean *(Uncle Ben's* Hearty*)*, ⅕ oz. 160
pea, green *(Cup-a-Soup)* 80
pea, split *(Aunt Patsy's Pantry)*, 3 tbsp. 160
pea, split *(Smart Soup)* 150
pea, split, w/carrots *(Health Valley)*, ½ cup 130
potato, w/broccoli *(Health Valley)*, ⅓ cup 70
potato cheese, w/ham *(Hormel* Micro Cup*)* 190
potato leek *(Smart Soup)* 120
rice and beans, red *(Smart Soup)* 180
tomato *(Cup-a-Soup)* 100
tomato basil *(Uncle Ben's* Hearty*)* 110
tomato rice Parmesano *(Fantastic)*, 1.9 oz. 200
tomato vegetable *(Campbell's Soupsations)* 130
vegetable *(Lipton Recipe Secrets)*, 1 cup* 30
vegetable *(Mrs. Grass Soup/Recipe)*, ¼ pkg. 35
vegetable, beef *(Mrs. Grass)*, ¼ pkg. 70
vegetable, chicken flavor *(Cup-a-Soup)* 50
vegetable, chicken flavor, creamy *(Cup-a-Soup)* 80
vegetable, spring *(Cup-a-Soup)* 45
Soup base, bottled *(Goya* Sofrito*)*, 1 tsp. 5

Soy beverage, 8 fl. oz.:
(EdenSoy/EdenSoy Extra) 130
(Soy Moo Fat Free) 110
carob *(EdenSoy)* 150
vanilla *(EdenSoy/EdenSoy* Extra) 150
Soy butter, roasted *(Natural Touch),* 2 tbsp. 170
Soy flour *(Arrowhead Mills),* ½ cup 200
Soy milk, see "Soy beverage"
Soy sauce, 1 tbsp.:
(Kikkoman/Kikkoman Light) 10
(La Choy/Chun King) 10
(La Choy Lite/*Chun King* Lite) 15
shoyu *(Eden* Natural/Organic) 15
tamari *(Eden* Domestic) 15
tamari *(Eden* Imported) 10
Soybeans, canned, black *(Eden* Organic), ½ cup 90
Soybeans, fermented, see "Miso" and "Natto"
Soybean cake or curd, see "Tofu"
Soybean kernels, roasted, toasted:
1 oz. or 95 kernels 129
whole, 1 cup 490
salted, whole, 1 cup 490
Soybean sprouts *(Jonathan's),* 1 cup, 3 oz. 100
Spaghetti, see "Pasta"
Spaghetti entree, canned, 1 cup:
w/franks *(Franco-American* SpaghettiO's) 250
w/meatballs *(Franco-American* SpaghettiO's/Superiore) . 260
tomato-cheese sauce *(Franco-American* SpaghettiO's) . 190
Spaghetti entree, frozen:
w/meat sauce *(Lean Cuisine),* 11.5 oz. 300
w/meat sauce *(Morton),* 8.5 oz. 200
w/meatballs *(Lean Cuisine),* 9.5 oz. 280
w/meatballs *(Stouffer's),* 12⅝ oz. 440
w/seasoned beef *(Healthy Choice),* 13.5 oz. 280
Spaghetti sauce, see "Pasta sauce"
Spaghetti squash, baked or boiled, drained, ½ cup 23
Spareribs, see "Pork" and "Pork, barbecued,
    refrigerated"
Spearmint, dried *(McCormick),* ¼ tsp. 1
Spelt flakes *(Arrowhead Mills),* 1 cup 100

Spelt flour *(Arrowhead Mills)*, ¼ cup 100
Spinach, fresh:
raw, chopped *(Dole)*, 1 cup 15
boiled, drained, ½ cup 21
Spinach, canned, ½ cup:
canned *(Popeye* Low Sodium) 35
canned *(S&W)* 30
canned, leaf *(Popeye)* 45
canned, leaf or chopped *(Del Monte)* 30
canned, chopped *(Popeye/Sunshine)* 40
Spinach, frozen, ½ cup, except as noted:
(Green Giant), ¾ cup 25
(Green Giant Harvest Fresh) 25
chopped *(Seabrook)*, ⅓ cup 20
in butter sauce, cut *(Green Giant)* 40
Spinach, water *(Frieda's* Ong Choy), 2 cups, 3 oz. 20
Spinach dip *(Marie's)*, 2 tbsp. 140
Spinach dishes, frozen:
creamed *(Green Giant)*, ½ cup 80
creamed *(Seabrook)*, ½ cup 120
creamed *(Stouffer's* Side Dish), ½ of 9-oz. pkg. 160
Indian *(Deep* Palak Paneer), 5 oz. 230
soufflé *(Stouffer's* Side Dish), 4 oz. 150
Spinach-feta pocket *(Amy's Pocketfuls)*, 1 piece 200
Spiny lobster, meat only:
boiled or steamed, 2-lb. lobster w/shell 233
boiled or steamed, 4 oz. 138
Spirals, pasta, canned, and chicken *(Libby's Diner)*,
  7¾ oz. 130
Split peas:
dry *(Goya)*, ¼ cup 110
boiled, ½ cup 116
Spot, meat only, baked or broiled, 4 oz. 179
Spring onion, see "Onion, green"
Sprouts (see also specific listings):
bean *(Frieda's)*, 1 oz. 10
bean, canned *(La Choy)*, 1 cup 10
hot and spicy *(Jonathan's)*, 1 cup, 4 oz. 25
mixed *(Shaw's)*, 2 oz. 9

Squash (see also specific squash listings):
canned *(Stokely)*, ½ cup 50
frozen *(Birds Eye)*, ½ cup 50
Squid:
meat only, raw, 4 oz. 104
canned *(Goya)*, ⅓ can 45
canned, in juice *(Goya)*, ¼ cup 120
Starfruit, see "Carambola"
Steak, see "Beef"
Steak sandwich, see "Beef sandwich"
Steak sauce, 1 tbsp.:
(A.1.) 15
(A.1. Bold) 20
(A.1. Thick and Hearty) 25
(Heinz 57) 15
(HP) 15
(Hunt's) 10
(Texas Best) 15
Caribbean style *(Tabasco)* 15
New Orleans style *(Tabasco)* 10
Stir-fry sauce (see also specific listings), 1 tbsp.:
(Ka•Me) 10
(Ken's Steak House) 20
(Kikkoman) 15
(Lawry's) 25
(S&W Oriental) 20
garlic and ginger *(Rice Road)* 25
honey *(Ken's Steak House)* 20
Strawberry:
fresh, ½ cup 23
canned, in light syrup *(Oregon)*, ½ cup 100
canned, whole, in syrup *(Comstock)*, ½ cup 140
frozen *(Big Valley)*, ⅔ cup 50
frozen *(Stilwell)*, ⅔ cup 50
Strawberry, dried *(Frieda's)*, ½ cup, 1.4 oz. . . . 150
Strawberry drink, 8 fl. oz.:
(Snapple Squeeze) 120
banana *(R.W. Knudsen)* 120
banana nectar *(Kern's)* 150
guava *(R.W. Knudsen)* 110

Strawberry drink *(cont.)*
kiwi *(R.W. Knudsen)* 120
kiwi *(Tropicana Twister)* 130
Strawberry juice, 8 fl. oz.:
(Veryfine Juice-Ups) 140
nectar *(R.W. Knudsen)* 120
Strawberry milk *(Nestlé Quik),* 1 cup 230
Strawberry milk drink mix *(Nestlé Quik),* 2 tbsp. 90
Strawberry syrup:
(Hershey's), 2 tbsp. 100
(R.W. Knudsen), ¼ cup 150
(S&W Reduced Calorie), ¼ cup 60
Strawberry topping, 2 tbsp.:
(Kraft) 110
(Smucker's) 100
Melba *(Dickinson's)* 90
String beans, see "Green beans"
Stroganoff gravy *(Pepperidge Farm),* ¼ cup 30
Stroganoff sauce, beef *(Lawry's),* 1 tbsp. 20
Stroganoff seasoning mix *(Durkee),* ⅛ pkg. 10
Stuffing (see also "Stuffing mix"):
(Arnold Unspiced), 2 cups 250
chicken, classic *(Pepperidge Farm),* ½ cup 130
corn bread *(Arnold/Brownberry),* 2 cups 250
country style or cube *(Pepperidge Farm),* ¾ cup 140
cube, bread, unseasoned *(Brownberry),* 2 cups 240
herb seasoned or sage-onion *(Arnold),* 2 cups 240
seasoned *(Arnold),* 2 cups 250
Stuffing mix, ⅙ pkg., except as noted:
all varieties *(Rice-A-Roni),* 1 cup* 170
all varieties *(Stove Top)* 110
chicken flavor *(Stove Top* Microwave) 130
corn bread, homestyle *(Stove Top* Microwave) 120
herb *(Stove Top* Flexible Serve), 1 oz. 120
Sturgeon, meat only:
baked, broiled, or microwaved, 4 oz. 153
smoked, 4 oz. 196
Subway, 1 serving, except as noted:
sandwiches, deli style:
    bologna 292

ham 234
roast beef 245
Subway Seafood & Crab 298
Subway Seafood & Crab, w/lite mayo 256
tuna 354
tuna, w/lite mayo 279
turkey 235
submarines, 6 :
  BLT, wheat 327
  BLT, white 311
  chicken breast, roasted, wheat 348
  chicken breast, roasted, white 332
  chicken taco, wheat 436
  chicken taco, white 421
  Classic Italian B.M.T., wheat 460
  Classic Italian B.M.T., white 445
  cold cut trio, wheat 378
  cold cut trio, white 362
  ham, wheat 302
  ham, white 287
  Italian, spicy, wheat 482
  Italian, spicy, white 467
  meatball, wheat 419
  meatball, white 404
  pizza sub, wheat 464
  pizza sub, white 448
  roast beef, wheat 303
  roast beef, white 288
  steak & cheese, wheat 398
  steak & cheese, white 383
  Subway Club, wheat 312
  Subway Club, white 297
  Subway Melt, wheat 382
  Subway Melt, white 366
  Subway Seafood & Crab, wheat 430
  Subway Seafood & Crab, wheat, w/lite mayo 347
  Subway Seafood & Crab, white 415
  Subway Seafood & Crab, white, w/lite mayo 332
  tuna, wheat 542
  tuna, wheat, w/lite mayo 391

Subway, submarines, 6 *(cont.)*
- tuna, white 527
- tuna, white, w/lite mayo 376
- turkey, wheat 289
- turkey, white 273
- turkey breast & ham, wheat 295
- turkey breast & ham, white 280
- *Veggie Delite,* wheat 237
- *Veggie Delite,* white 222

salads:
- BLT 140
- chicken breast, roasted 162
- chicken taco 250
- *Classic Italian B.M.T.* 274
- cold cut trio 191
- ham 116
- meatball 233
- pizza 277
- roast beef 117
- steak & cheese 212
- *Subway Club* 126
- *Subway Melt* 195
- *Subway Seafood & Crab* 244
- *Subway Seafood & Crab,* w/lite mayo 161
- tuna 356
- tuna, w/lite mayo 205
- turkey breast 102
- turkey breast & ham 109
- *Veggie Delite* 51

salad dressings, 1 tbsp.:
- French, creamy Italian, or Thousand Island 65
- French, fat free 15
- Italian, fat free 5
- ranch 87
- ranch, fat free 12

standard fixin's, onions, lettuce, tomatoes, pickle chips, pepper strips, olive rings, or onions, average
- serving . . . . <5

condiments:
- bacon, 2 slices 45

cheese, 2 triangles 41
mayonnaise dressing, 1 tsp. 37
mayonnaise dressing, lite, 1 tsp. 18
mustard, 2 tsp. 8
olive oil blend, 1 tsp. 45
vinegar, 1 tsp. 1
cookies, 1.3-oz. piece:
   Brazil nut & chocolate chips or sugar 230
   chocolate chip, chunk, or *M&M's* 210
   oatmeal raisin 200
   peanut butter 220
   white chip macadamia nut 230
Succotash, canned, ½ cup:
whole kernel *(S&W)* 100
whole kernel *(Seneca)* 90
Sucker, white, meat only, baked or broiled, 4 oz. 135
Sugar, beet or cane:
brown, light or dark *(Domino)*, 1 tsp. 15
granulated, 1 tbsp. 46
granulated, 1 tsp. 15
powdered or confectioners', 1 cup, sifted 389
powdered or confectioners', 1 tbsp., unsifted 31
Sugar, substitute *(Sweet 'n Low)*, 1 pkt. 4
Sugar apple, 1 medium, 9.9 oz. 146
Sugar loaf squash *(Frieda's)*, ¾ cup, 3 oz. 30
Sugar snap peas, see "Peas, edible-podded"
Summer sausage:
(Old Smokehouse), 1 oz. 110
beef *(Oscar Mayer)*, 2 slices, 1.6 oz. 140
Sunfish, pumpkinseed, meat only, baked or broiled,
   4 oz. 129
Sunflower seeds:
(Frito-Lay), 1 oz. 180
barbecued kernels *(Planters)*, 1.7 oz. 290
dry-roasted, in shell *(Planters)*, ¾ cup, 1 oz. edible 160
dry-roasted, kernels *(Planters)*, ¼ cup 190
honey-roasted, kernels *(Planters)*, 1.7 oz. 280
oil-roasted, kernels *(Planters)*, 2 oz. 340
salted kernels *(Planters)*, 1 oz. 170
tamari-roasted *(Eden)*, 1 oz. 170

Sunflower seed butter *(Roaster Fresh)*, 1 oz. 160
Swamp cabbage, boiled, drained, chopped, ½ cup 10
Sweet potato:
raw *(Dole)*, 1 medium, 4.6 oz. 130
baked in skin, 1 medium 118
baked in skin, mashed, ½ cup 103
Sweet potato, canned:
(Seneca Yams), ½ cup 150
whole *(Royal Prince/Trappey's)*, 4 pieces 200
whole *(Royal Prince* 9 oz.), 3 pieces 200
cut *(Allens/Sugary Sam/Princella* Yams), ⅔ cup 160
halves *(Royal Prince)*, 3 pieces 190
mashed *(Princella/Sugary Sam)*, ⅔ cup 120
candied or orange-pineapple *(Royal Prince)*, ½ cup 210
candied *(S&W)*, ½ cup 170
Sweet potato, frozen, candied:
(Mrs. Paul's), 5 fl. oz. 300
(Mrs. Paul's Sweets'n Apples), 1¼ cups 270
(Ore-Ida), 5 pieces 170
Sweet potato chips *(Terra* Chips), 1 oz. 140
Sweet and sour sauce, 2 tbsp.:
(Ka•Me) 50
(Kikkoman) 35
(La Choy/Chun King) 60
(Sauceworks) 60
(Woody's) 70
(World Harbors Maui Mountain) 60
duck sauce *(Ka•Me)* 80
duck sauce *(La Choy)* 60
Sweetbreads, see "Pancreas" and "Thymus"
Swiss chard:
raw *(Frieda's)*, 1 cup, 3 oz. 15
boiled, drained, chopped, ½ cup 18
Swiss steak gravy mix *(Durkee)*, ¼ cup* 15
Swordfish, meat only:
fresh, baked or broiled, 4 oz. 176
frozen, steaks *(Peter Pan)*, 4 oz. 160
Syrup, see specific listings
Szechwan sauce *(Ka•Me)*, 1 tbsp. 20

FOOD AND MEASURE	CALORIES

Tabouli *(Frieda's)*, ½ cup	152
Tabouli mix *(Fantastic)*, ¼ cup	120

Taco Bell, 1 serving:

breakfast items:

burrito, bacon and egg, double	480
burrito, country	270
burrito, fiesta	280
burrito, grande	420
quesadilla, cheese	380
quesadilla w/bacon	450
quesadilla w/sausage	430

burritos:

bacon cheeseburger	570
bean	380
Big Beef Burrito Supreme	520
Big Chicken Burrito Supreme	510
Burrito Supreme	440
chicken, grilled	410
chicken club	540
chili cheese	330
7 layer	530

Border Wraps:

chicken *Fajita Wrap*	470
chicken *Fajita Wrap* Supreme	520
steak *Fajita Wrap*	470
steak *Fajita Wrap* Supreme	510
veggie *Fajita Wrap*	420
veggie *Fajita Wrap* Supreme	470

tacos:

BLT soft taco	340
Double Decker taco	340
Double Decker Taco Supreme	390
grilled chicken soft taco	240

Taco Bell, tacos (cont.)

grilled steak soft taco	230
grilled steak soft *Taco Supreme*	290
soft taco	220
soft *Taco Supreme*	260
steak soft taco	200
taco	180
Taco Supreme	220

specialty items:

Big Beef MexiMelt	290
Mexican pizza	570
quesadilla, cheese	350
quesadilla, chicken	410
taco salad w/salsa	850
taco salad w/salsa, w/out shell	420
tostada	300

nachos and sides:

Big Beef Nachos Supreme	450
cinnamon twists	140
Mexican rice	190
nachos	320
nachos *BellGrande*	770
pintos 'n cheese	190

sauces and condiments:

cheese, cheddar	30
cheese, pepper jack	25
green sauce or pico de gallo	5
guacamole	35
nacho cheese sauce	120
picante or taco sauce	0
red sauce	10
salsa	25
sour cream	40

Taco mix, dinner, 2 tacos*, except as noted:

(Lawry's), ⅕ pkg.	150
(Old El Paso/Las Palmas)	270
nacho cheese *(Old El Paso One Skillet Mexican)*	490
salsa flavor *(Old El Paso One Skillet Mexican)*	460
soft *(Old El Paso)*	380
taco flavor *(Old El Paso One Skillet Mexican)*	440

Taco sauce:
(Hunt's Manwich), ¼ cup 30
(Lawry's Chunky), 2 tbsp. 10
(Lawry's Sauce'n Seasoner), 2 tbsp. 15
(Pancho Villa), 2 tbsp. 15
all varieties *(Old El Paso)*, 1 tbsp. 5
Taco seasoning mix:
(Durkee Pouch), ⅛ pkg. 15
(Lawry's), 1 tbsp. 25
(Old El Paso/Las Palmas), 2 tsp. 20
(Old El Paso 40% Less Sodium), 2 tsp. 15
chicken *(Lawry's)*, 2 tsp. 20
salad *(Durkee* Pouch), ⅙ pkg. 20
salad *(Lawry's)*, 1 tsp. 15
Taco shell:
(Gebhardt), 3 shells 155
(Las Palmas), 3 shells 180
(Lawry's), 2 shells 120
(Lawry's Super Size), 2 shells 180
(Old El Paso Super), 2 shells 200
(Rosarita), 3 shells 155
golden *(Old El Paso)*, 3 shells 170
mini *(Old El Paso)*, 7 shells 170
soft, see "Tortilla"
tostada *(Rosarita)*, 2 shells 125
tostada or white corn *(Old El Paso)*, 3 shells 170
Tahini *(Krinos)*, 2 tbsp. 260
Tamale, canned:
(Gebhardt), 2 pieces 270
(Gebhardt Jumbo), 2 pieces 330
(Van Camp), 2 pieces 210
beef *(Hormel)*, 3 pieces 280
beef, jumbo *(Hormel)*, 2 pieces 270
chicken *(Hormel)*, 3 pieces 210
in chili gravy *(Old El Paso)*, ½ can 320
Tamale pie, Mexican, frozen *(Amy's)*, 8 oz. 220
Tamari, see "Soy sauce"
Tamarillo:
red *(Frieda's)*, 2 pieces, 4¼ oz. 40
yellow *(Frieda's)*, 2 pieces, 4¼ oz. 30

Tamarind, 1 fruit, 3 ∞1 5
Tandoori paste, mild *(Patak's),* 2 tbsp. 30
Tangerine:
fresh *(Dole),* 2 fruits 70
canned, in juice *(S&W* Mandarin), ⅔ cup 70
canned, in light syrup *(Del Monte* Mandarin), ½ cup . . . 80
canned, in light syrup *(Dole),* ½ cup 80
canned, in light syrup *(Haddon House* Clementines),
 ½ cup 80
Tangerine juice, 8 fl. oz.:
blend *(Dole* Mandarin) 140
blend *(Tropicana* Pure Premium) 110
blend *(Tropicana* Twister) 130
Tapioca, dry *(Minute),* 1½ tsp. 20
Tapioca pudding, see "Pudding"
Taro, cooked *(Frieda's),* 5 oz. 150
Taro chips, spiced *(Terra),* 1 oz. 130
Taro root, cooked *(Frieda's),* 5 oz. 150
Tarragon, dried *(McCormick),* ¼ tsp. 1
Tart shell, see "Pastry shell, frozen"
Tartar sauce, 2 tbsp.:
(Bookbinder's) 120
(Hellmann's/Best Foods) 140
(Hellmann's/Best Foods Low Fat) 40
lemon herb flavor *(Sauceworks)* 150
Tea, black, green, or herbal, all varieties *(Lipton Brisk/*
 Iced Tea Brew), 1 bag or tsp. 0
Tea, iced, 8 fl. oz., except as noted:
(Lipton's Iced Sweetened) 70
(Snapple Sweetened) 70
(Veryfine Chillers) 80
all fruit flavors *(Apple & Eve)* 100
all fruit flavors *(Lipton* Chilled) 80
Caribbean cooler *(Lipton Brisk),* 12 fl. oz. 130
ginseng or orange jasmine herbal *(Snapple)* 80
green *(Snapple)* 100
green tea and passion fruit *(Lipton's Iced)* 80
lemon *(Lipton Brisk* Chilled Original/Sweetened) 80
lemon *(Lipton's Iced)* 90
lemon, peach, or raspberry *(Snapple)* 100

mint *(Snapple)* 110
peach *(Lipton Brisk* Chilled) 80
peach or raspberry *(Lipton's Iced)* 110
raspberry *(Lipton Brisk* Chilled) 80
southern style, lemon flavor *(Lipton's Iced)* 100
tangerine twist *(Lipton Brisk)*, 12 fl. oz. 120
Teff seed or flour *(Arrowhead Mills)*, 2 oz. 200
Tempeh, 1 oz. 56
Tempura batter mix *(Golden Dipt)*, ¼ cup 120
Teriyaki sauce, 1 tbsp.:
(Chun King/Chun King Hot) 15
(La Choy/La Choy Lite) 20
baste and glaze *(Kikkoman)* 50
baste and glaze, w/honey and pineapple *(Kikkoman)* . . . 80
cooking, and marinade *(S&W/S&W* Lite) 25
marinade *(Lawry's)* 20
marinade and *(Kikkoman)* 15
marinade and *(Lea & Perrins)* 15
Teriyaki seasoning mix, beef *(Durkee)*, 1 tbsp. 30
Thai pepper *(Frieda's)*, 1 piece, 1.1 oz. 10
Thai sauce *(World Harbors* Nong Khai), 2 tbsp. 40
Thyme, dried *(McCormick)*, ¼ tsp. 4
Thymus:
beef, braised, 4 oz. 362
veal, braised, 4 oz. 197
Tilefish, meat only, baked or broiled, 4 oz. 167
Tofu:
fresh, extra firm *(Nasoya)*, ⅕ of 1-lb. block 90
fresh, firm *(Frieda's)*, 3 oz. 60
fresh, firm *(Nasoya)*, ⅕ of 1-lb. block 80
fresh, silken *(Nasoya)*, ⅕ of 1-lb. block 50
fresh, soft *(Nasoya)*, ⅙ of 1-lb. block 60
5-spice or French *(Nasoya)*, ¼ block 70
Tofu seasoning mix: all varieties, except Mandarin and
    Szechwan stir-fry *(TofuMate)*, ¼ pkg. 15
breakfast scramble *(Fantastic* Classics), 2½ tbsp. 60
Mandarin stir-fry *(TofuMate)*, ¼ pkg. 30
Szechwan stir-fry *(TofuMate)*, ¼ pkg. 25
Tom Collins mixer, bottled *(Holland House)*, 3 fl. oz. . 160
Tomatillo, in jars *(La Victoria* Entero), 5 pieces 40

Tomato:

raw, 2³/₅ -diam. tomato 26
raw, chopped, ½ cup 19
boiled, ½ cup 32
Tomato, canned (see also "Tomato sauce"), ½ cup,
   except as noted:
whole *(Del Monte)* 25
whole *(Hunt's/Hunt's* No Salt), 2 pieces 20
whole, Italian pear, w/basil *(S&W)* 25
whole, peeled *(Progresso)* 20
whole, peeled *(S&W)* 25
whole, peeled *(S&W* No Salt) 20
chunky, chili style *(Del Monte)* 30
chunky, pasta style *(Del Monte)* 45
crushed *(Hunt's/Hunt's* Angela Mia) 30
crushed *(Progresso)*, ¼ cup 20
crushed *(S&W)*, ¼ cup 20
cut *(Hunt's* Choice Cut) 20
cut, in juice *(S&W* Ready-Cut/Ready-Cut No Salt) . . . 25
cut, in puree *(S&W* Ready-Cut) 30
diced *(Del Monte/Del Monte* No Salt) 25
diced, w/basil, garlic, oregano *(Del Monte)* 50
diced, w/Italian herbs or garlic *(Hunt's* Choice Cut) . . . 25
diced, w/onion, garlic *(Del Monte)* 35
paste or puree, see "Tomato paste" and "Tomato
   puree"
primavera *(Contadina* Pasta Ready) 50
stewed *(Del Monte/Del Monte* No Salt) 35
stewed *(Hunt's/Hunt's* No Salt) 35
stewed, Italian *(Del Monte)* 30
stewed, Italian *(Green Giant)* 30
stewed, Mexican *(Green Giant)* 35
stewed, Mexican or Cajun *(Del Monte)* 35
Tomato, dried:
(Frieda's No Salt), 1 oz. 86
flakes *(Christopher Ranch)*, 3 tbsp. 80
julienne *(Sonoma)*, 7–9 strips 15
seasoning *(Sonoma* Season It), 2–3 tsp. 20
Tomato, green, fresh, 2³/₅ -diam. tomato 30
Tomato, pickled *(Claussen)*, 1 oz. 5

Tomato, sun-dried, see "Tomato, dried"

Tomato dip, sun-dried *(Marie's)*, 2 tbsp. 140

Tomato juice, 8 fl. oz., except as noted:

(Campbell's/Campbell's Healthy Request) 50

(Del Monte) 50

(Del Monte Not from Concentrate) 40

(Hunt's) 20

(Hunt's No Salt) 35

(S&W) 40

(Sacramento) 35

Tomato paste, all varieties *(Hunt's)*, 2 tbsp. 30

Tomato puree *(Hunt's)*, ¼ cup 25

Tomato sauce (see also "Pasta sauce"), ¼ cup:

(Del Monte/Del Monte No Salt) 20

(Hunt's/Hunt's No Salt) 15

(Progresso) 20

chili, chunky *(Hunt's Ready Sauce)* 20

chunky *(Hunt's Ready Sauce)* 15

chunky Mexican *(Hunt's Ready Sauce* Special) 20

garden, original or Mexican *(S&W)* 20

garlic *(Hunt's Ready Sauce)* 30

garlic and herb *(Hunt's Ready Sauce)* 25

herb, country *(Hunt's Ready Sauce)* 35

Italian *(Hunt's/Hunt's Ready Sauce)* 30

Italian, chunky *(Hunt's Ready Sauce)* 25

meat loaf *(Hunt's Ready Sauce Meatloaf Fixin's)* 20

salsa *(Hunt's Ready Sauce* Special) 20

w/green chilies or jalapeños *(Old El Paso)* 10

Tomato tapenade, dried *(Sonoma)*, 1 tbsp. 70

Tomato-beef cocktail *(Beefamato)*, 8 fl. oz. 80

Tomato-chili cocktail *(Snap-E-Tom)*, 6 fl. oz. 40

Tomato-clam cocktail *(Clamato)*, 8 fl. oz. 100

Tongue, braised, beef, 4 oz. 321

Tongue lunch meat, beef *(Hebrew National)*, 2 oz. 120

Tortellini (see also "Tortelloni"):

cheese *(Di Giorno)*, ¾ cup 260

cheese, herb and garlic *(Real Torino)*, 1 cup 320

cheese, three *(Contadina)*, ¾ cup 250

chicken *(Real Torino)*, 1 cup 300

chicken, herb *(Contadina)*, ¾ cup 260

Tortellini *(cont.)*
spinach *(Putney)*, 1 cup 290
tofu *(Soy-Boy)*, 7/8 cup 190
Tortellini dish, frozen, cheese *(The Budget Gourmet
  Side Dish)*, 6.25 oz. 190
Tortellini entree, canned:
cheese *(Chef Boyardee)*, 1 cup 230
ground beef *(Chef Boyardee)*, 7½ oz. 220
meat *(Chef Boyardee)*, 1 cup 260
Tortelloni, refrigerated, 1 cup, except as noted:
cheese, dried tomato *(Real Torino Sanoma)* 310
cheese, four *(Real Torino)* 310
w/chicken and herbs *(Di Giorno)* 260
hot red pepper and cheese *(Di Giorno)* 310
mozzarella garlic *(Di Giorno)* 300
mushroom *(Di Giorno)* 290
pumpkin *(Tutta Pasta)*, 11 pieces, 3.2 oz. 210
sausage *(Contadina)* 320
Tortilla, 1 piece, except as noted:
(Cedar's Boston), 1.1-oz. piece 100
(Cedar's Boston), 2.6-oz. piece 200
flour *(Goya)* 110
flour *(Mesa 6)* 80
flour *(Old El Paso)* 140
flour, small *(Goya)* 80
flour, frozen *(Tyson)*, 1.9 oz. 170
flour, heat pressed *(Tyson)*, 2 pieces 180
soft taco *(Old El Paso)*, 2 pieces 170
soft taco, refrigerated *(Old El Paso)* 110
Tortilla chips, see "Corn chips, puffs, and similar
  snacks"
Tostaco or tostada shell, see "Taco shell"
Trail mix:
(Sonoma), ¼ cup 160
California *(Dole)*, 1.2 oz. 130
Hawaiian *(Dole)*, 1.2 oz. 150
Sierra *(Del Monte)*, 1 oz. 120
Tree fern, cooked, chopped, ½ cup 28
Trout, meat only, 4 oz.:
mixed species, baked or broiled 215

rainbow, farmed, baked or broiled 192
rainbow, wild, baked or broiled 170
sea, see "Sea trout"
Tuna, meat only, 4 oz.:
bluefin, baked or broiled 209
skipjack, baked or broiled 150
yellowfin, baked or broiled 158
yellowtail, frozen *(Peter Pan)* 110
Tuna, canned, drained, 2 oz.:
chunk light, in oil *(Chicken of the Sea)* 110
chunk light, in oil *(S&W)* 110
chunk light, in oil *(StarKist)* 110
chunk light, in water *(S&W)* 70
chunk light, fillet, or white, in water *(StarKist)* 60
solid, olive oil *(Progresso)* 160
solid white, in oil *(Chicken of the Sea)* 90
solid white, in oil *(S&W)* 80
solid white, in oil *(StarKist)* 90
solid white, in water *(StarKist)* 70
"Tuna," vegetarian, frozen *(Worthington Tuno)*, ½ cup . . 80
Tuna entree, frozen, and noodles:
(Stouffer's Casserole), 10 oz. 320
(Swanson Lunch and More Casserole), 1 pkg. 320
(Weight Watchers Casserole), 9.5 oz. 270
chunky *(Marie Callender)*, 12 oz. 960
Tuna entree mix, 1 cup*:
au gratin, creamy broccoli, cheddar, fettuccine Alfredo,
  or tetrazzini *(Tuna Helper)* 310
melt *(Tuna Helper)* 300
pasta, cheesy *(Tuna Helper)* 280
pasta, creamy *(Tuna Helper)* 300
pasta salad *(Tuna Helper)* 380
potpie *(Tuna Helper)* 440
Romanoff *(Tuna Helper)* 280
Tuna spread:
(Underwood), ¼ cup 50
salad *(Bumble Bee)*, 2.75-oz. can 70
salad *(Libby's Spreadables)*, ⅓ cup 130
Turban squash *(Frieda's)*, ¾ cup, 3 oz. 30
Turbot, European, meat only, baked or broiled, 4 oz. . . . 138

Turkey (see also "Turkey, frozen or refrigerated"),
  fresh, roasted, 4 oz., except as noted:

meat w/skin 236
meat only 193
meat only, diced, 1 cup 238
skin only, 1 oz. 125
dark meat, w/skin 251
dark meat, meat only 212
dark meat, meat only, diced, 1 cup 262
light meat, w/skin 223
light meat, meat only 178
light meat, meat only, diced, 1 cup 219
back, meat w/skin 276
breast, meat w/skin, ½ breast, 1.9 lb. (4.2 lb. raw
  w/bone) 1,637
breast, meat w/skin 214
leg, meat w/skin, 1 leg, 1.2 lb. (1.5 lb. raw w/bone) . . 1,133
leg, meat w/skin 236
wing, meat w/skin, 1 wing, 6.6 oz. (9.9 oz. raw
  w/bone) 426
wing, meat w/skin 260
Turkey, canned, chunk, 2 oz.:
(Hormel) 70
white *(Hormel)* 60
Turkey, frozen or refrigerated:
whole, cooked:
  dark meat, hen *(Perdue)*, 3 oz. 180
  dark meat, tom *(Perdue)*, 3 oz. 160
  white meat, hen *(Perdue)*, 3 oz. 150
  white meat, tom *(Perdue)*, 3 oz. 140
  barbecued *(Empire* Kosher), 5 oz. 250
breast, cooked:
  (Perdue Whole or Half), 3 oz. 150
  boneless *(Perdue Fit 'n Easy)*, 3 oz. 110
  cutlets, thin sliced *(Perdue Fit 'n Easy)*, 2.4 oz. 90
  oven roasted *(Hebrew National)*, 2 oz. 60
breast, smoked *(Hebrew National)*, 2 oz. 60
breast, smoked *(Hormel Light & Lean* 97), 3 oz. 80
drumstick, cooked *(Perdue)*, 3 oz. 130
ground, see "Turkey, ground"

maple glaze *(Boar's Head Honey Coat)*, 3 oz. 100
roast, boneless *(Norbest)*, 4 oz. 135
smoked, hickory *(Norbest Young)*, 3 oz. 145
thigh, cooked *(Perdue)*, 3 oz. 190
wing, cooked *(Perdue/Perdue Tom/Portions)*, 3 oz. . . . 160
wing, roasted *(Perdue Drummettes)*, 3.3-oz. piece 180
Turkey, ground:
raw *(Louis Rich)*, 4 oz. 190
raw, breast *(Perdue)*, 4 oz. 120
raw, 85% lean *(Shady Brook Farms)*, 4 oz. 220
raw, meat loaf *(Shady Brook Farms)*, 4 oz. 150
raw, patty, white *(Louis Rich)*, 4 oz. 150
cooked *(Perdue/Perdue Burgers)*, 3 oz. 160
cooked, breast *(Perdue)*, 3 oz. 110
"Turkey," vegetarian:
canned *(Worthington Turkee)*, 3 slices 190
Turkey bacon *(Louis Rich)*, .5-oz. slice 30
Turkey bologna *(Louis Rich)*, 1-oz. slice 50
Turkey dinner, frozen:
breast *(Healthy Choice)*, 10.5 oz. 290
breast, w/pasta *(Swanson)*, 1 pkg. 270
and gravy, dressing *(Banquet Extra Helping)*, 17 oz. . . . 630
and gravy, dressing *(Freezer Queen Meal)*, 9.2 oz. 210
roast, country *(Healthy Choice)*, 10 oz. 250
white meat, mostly *(Swanson)*, 1 pkg. 320
white meat, mostly *(Swanson Hungry-Man)*, 1 pkg. 510
Turkey entree, canned:
gravy and dressing *(Libby's Diner)*, 7 oz. 180
stew *(Dinty Moore)*, 1 cup 150
Turkey entree, frozen:
(Lean Cuisine Homestyle), 9³⁄₈ oz. 240
breast, honey roast *(Banquet)*, 9 oz. 270
breast, stuffed *(Weight Watchers)*, 9 oz. 230
glazed *(Lean Cuisine Cafe Classics)*, 9 oz. 250
and gravy, dressing *(Freezer Queen Homestyle)*, 9 oz. . 210
gravy and, sliced *(Banquet Family)*, 2 slices w/gravy . . . 150
gravy and, sliced *(Banquet Toppers)*, 5-oz. bag 160
gravy and, w/dressing *(Morton)*, 9 oz. 230
grilled breast and rice pilaf *(Marie Callender)*, 11³⁄₄ oz. . 320
pie *(Banquet)*, 7-oz. pie 370

Turkey entree, frozen *(cont.)*
pie *(Marie Callender)*, 9.5-oz. pie 610
pie *(Stouffer's)*, 10-oz. pie 530
pie *(Swanson)*, 1 pkg. 400
pie *(Swanson Hungry-Man)*, 1 pkg. 650
roast, breast, and stuffing *(Lean Cuisine)*, 9¾ oz. 290
roast, w/mushrooms *(Healthy Choice)*, 8.5 oz. 230
roast, and stuffing *(Stouffer's Homestyle)*, 9⅝ oz. 320
white meat, mostly *(Banquet)*, 9¼ oz. 280
white meat, mostly *(Swanson Lunch and More)*, 1 pkg. . 240
Turkey frankfurter, 1 link:
(Empire Kosher) 90
and chicken *(Louis Rich 8 links, 12 oz.)*, 1.5 oz. 80
and chicken *(Louis Rich 10 links, 16 oz.)*, 1.6 oz. 90
and chicken *(Louis Rich Bun-Length)* 110
Turkey giblets, simmered, chopped or diced, 1 cup . . . 243
Turkey gravy, ¼ cup:
canned *(Franco-American)* 25
canned *(Franco-American Fat Free)* 20
canned, roasted *(Heinz)* 25
canned, slow-roasted *(Franco-American)* 30
mix* *(Durkee/French's)* 20
mix*, roasted *(Knorr)* 25
Turkey ham:
(Healthy Deli), 2 oz. 70
(Louis Rich), 1-oz. slice 30
(Louis Rich Deli-Thin), 4 slices, 2 oz. 60
canned *(Hormel)*, 2 oz. 70
honey cured *(Louis Rich)*, 1-oz. slice 70
Turkey hash, canned roast *(Mary Kitchen)*, 1 cup 210
Turkey lunch meat (see also "Turkey ham," etc.),
  2 oz.:
(Boar's Head Ovengold/Ovengold Skinless/Salsalito) 60
(Hormel Deli Premium/Hormel Light & Lean 97) 50
(Hormel Sandwich Maker) 45
barbecued *(Louis Rich)* 60
Black Forest *(Healthy Deli)* 60
browned or smoked skinless *(Healthy Choice)* 50
champagne glazed, honey cured *(Black Bear)* 70
cured *(Norbest Gourmet)* 70

honey roasted, salsa, or Southwest *(Healthy Choice)* 60
honey roasted *(Healthy Deli)* 60
honey roasted *(Louis Rich)* 60
maple honey *(Boar's Head)* 70
oven roasted *(Black Bear* Catering Style) 50
oven roasted *(Healthy Choice)* 45
oven roasted *(Healthy Deli)* 60
oven roasted, Italian *(Healthy Deli)* 70
oven roasted or rotisserie flavor *(Louis Rich)* 50
skinless *(Hormel/Hormel* Deli) 50
smoked *(Boar's Head* Hickory) 70
smoked *(Boar's Head Cracked Pepper Mill)* 60
smoked *(Healthy Deli* Mesquite) 60
smoked *(Hebrew National* Hickory) 60
smoked, hickory *(Louis Rich)* 50
Tex-Mex *(Black Bear)* 60
Turkey pastrami, 2 oz.:
(Boar's Head) 60
(Healthy Deli) 70
(Louis Rich Chunk) 60
Turkey patty, breaded *(Louis Rich),* 1 piece 220
Turkey pie, see "Turkey entree"
Turkey salami:
(Louis Rich), 1-oz. slice 45
(Norbest), 2 oz. 85
cotto *(Louis Rich),* 1-oz. slice 40
Turkey sandwich, frozen, 1 piece:
w/broccoli and cheese *(Lean Pockets)* 260
and ham w/cheese *(Hot Pockets)* 320
and ham w/cheese *(Lean Pockets)* 270
and vegetables *(Healthy Choice Hearty Handfuls)* 320
Turkey sausage, uncooked, except as noted:
(Shady Brook Farms Old World), 4 oz. 190
breakfast *(Shady Brook Farms),* 4 oz. 80
breakfast, raw or cooked *(Perdue),* 2 links, 2 oz. 100
Italian, hot/sweet *(Louis Rich),* 2.5 oz. 120
Italian, hot/sweet *(Perdue),* 2.7-oz. link 110
Italian, hot/sweet *(Shady Brook Farms),* 4 oz. 170
Italian, hot/sweet, cooked *(Perdue),* 2.4-oz. link 110
smoked *(Louis Rich/Louis Rich* Polska), 2 oz. 90

Turkey sausage *(cont.)*
smoked, and duck, cooked *(Gerhard's Sausage)*,
2.5 oz. 100
Turkey spread:
chunky *(Underwood)*, ¼ cup 110
salad *(Libby's Spreadables)*, ⅓ cup 150
Turmeric, dried *(McCormick)*, ¼ tsp. 2
Turnip, fresh or stored:
boiled, drained, cubed, ½ cup 14
boiled, drained, mashed, ½ cup 21
Turnip greens, ½ cup:
fresh, boiled, drained, chopped 15
canned *(Allens/Sunshine)* 25
canned, chopped, w/diced turnips *(Allens/Sunshine)* . . . 30
frozen, w/diced turnips *(Seabrook)* 30
Turnover, apple *(Pillsbury)*, 2 pieces 350
Twists, pasta, canned, w/meat sauce *(Franco-American
Superiore)*, 1 cup 250
Tzatziki dip *(Western Creamy)*, 2 tbsp. 60

V

Vanilla shake (Nestlé Quik), 9 oz. 280
Veal, meat only, 4 oz.:
cubed, lean only, braised or stewed 213
ground, broiled 195
leg, braised, lean w/fat 239
leg, braised, lean only 230
leg, roasted, lean w/fat 181
leg, roasted, lean only 170
loin, braised, lean w/fat 322
loin, braised, lean only 256
loin, roasted, lean w/fat 246
loin, roasted, lean only 198
rib, braised, lean w/fat 285
rib, braised, lean only 247
rib, roasted, lean w/fat 259
rib, roasted, lean only 201
shoulder, whole, braised, lean w/fat 259
shoulder, whole, braised, lean only 226
shoulder, whole, roasted, lean w/fat 209
shoulder, whole, roasted, lean only 193
sirloin, braised, lean w/fat 286
sirloin, braised, lean only 231
sirloin, roasted, lean w/fat 229
sirloin, roasted, lean only 191
"Veal," vegetarian (Worthington Veelets), 1 patty . . . 180
Veal parmigiana dinner, frozen:
(Freezer Queen Meal), 10.2 oz. 290
(Swanson), 1 pkg. 440
(Swanson Hungry-Man), 1 pkg. 640
Veal parmigiana entree, frozen:
(Banquet), 9 oz. 360
(Morton), 8.75 oz. 280
w/spaghetti (Stouffer's Homestyle), 11⅞ oz. 430

Vegetable antipasto, in jars *(Paesana)*, 3¾ oz. 260
Vegetable burger, see " 'Hamburger,' vegetarian"
Vegetable curry, in jars *(Patak's)*, ½ cup 180
Vegetable dinner, frozen:
(Amy's Country), 11 oz. 380
loaf *(Amy's)*, 10 oz. 260
Vegetable entree, frozen:
country, and beef *(Lean Cuisine)*, 9 oz. 220
dumplings, in curry sauce *(Deep* Kofta Curry), 5 oz. . . . 245
pie *(Amy's)*, 7.5 oz. 360
pie *(Amy's* Nondairy), 7.5 oz. 320
pie, w/beef *(Morton)*, 7 oz. 340
pie, w/broccoli and cheese *(Tyson)*, 8.9-oz. pie 210
pie, w/cheese *(Banquet)*, 7-oz. pie 340
pie, w/chicken *(Morton)*, 7 oz. 320
pie, w/turkey *(Morton)*, 7 oz. 310
pie, shepherd's *(Amy's* Nondairy), 8 oz. 160
pilaf, Indian *(Deep)*, 1 cup 230
Vegetable entree mix, dry, stew *(Knorr)*, 1 pkg. 160
Vegetable juice, 8 fl. oz., except as noted:
(Campbell's V-8 Low Sodium) 60
(Campbell's V-8 100% *V-8* 100% *Healthy Request)* 50
(Hunt's Cocktail) 20
all flavors *(R.W. Knudsen Very Veggie)* 50
blend *(Dole)*, 12 fl. oz. 90
picante or spicy hot *(Campbell's V-8* 100%) 50
spicy *(Dole)*, 12 fl. oz. 80
tangy, lightly *(Campbell's V-8* 100%) 60
Vegetable oyster, see "Salsify"
Vegetable pie, see "Vegetable entree"
Vegetables, see specific listings
Vegetables, mixed, fresh:
Asian stir-fry *(Frieda's)*, 3 oz. 15
California or garden style *(Dole)*, 3 oz. 30
Chinese, fancy *(La Choy)*, ⅔ cup 9
chop suey *(La Choy)*, ½ cup 10
chow mein *(Chun King)*, ⅔ cup 15
Italian style *(Dole)*, 3 oz. 25
New England *(Dole)*, 3 oz. 50
Oriental style *(Dole)*, 3 oz. 30

Vegetables, mixed, canned, ½ cup:
(Del Monte/Del Monte No Salt) 40
(Green Giant) 60
(Green Giant Garden Medley) 40
(S&W) 35
(Stokely/Stokely No Salt) 35
regular or for stew *(Seneca)* 45
and sauce *(House of Tsang* Cantonese/Szechuan) 70
and sauce, sweet and sour *(House of Tsang* Hong
    Kong) 160
and sauce teriyaki *(House of Tsang* Tokyo) 100
stew *(Stokely)* 45
Vegetables, mixed, frozen:
(Green Giant), ¾ cup 50
(Green Giant Harvest Fresh), ⅔ cup 50
(Seneca), ⅔ cup 60
Bavarian, w/spaetzle/bacon bits *(Birds Eye),* 1 cup 150
in butter sauce *(Green Giant),* ¾ cup 70
French style, in herb butter sauce *(Birds Eye),* ⅔ cup . 110
Italian style, in garlic basil sauce *(Birds Eye),* 1 cup . . . 150
Oriental blend or stir-fry *(Seneca),* ¾ cup 25
Scandinavian blend or soup mix *(Seneca),* ¾ cup 40
stir-fry, in seasoned soy sauce *(Birds Eye),* ½ cup 60
winter blend *(Seneca),* 1 cup 25
Vegetables, mixed, pickled *(Zorba),* ½ cup 20
Vegetarian burger, see " 'Hamburger,' vegetarian"
Vegetarian entree (see also specific listings):
canned *(Loma Linda Swiss Stake),* 1 piece 120
canned *(Worthington Numete),* ⅜ slice 130
canned *(Worthington Protose),* ⅜ slice 130
canned, choplet *(Worthington),* 2 pieces 90
canned, cutlet *(Worthington),* 1 piece 70
canned, cuts, dinner *(Loma Linda),* 2 pieces 90
canned, multigrain *(Worthington* 20 oz.), 2 pieces 100
frozen *(Worthington FriPats),* 1 patty 130
frozen *(Worthington Stakelets),* 1 piece 140
frozen, croquettes *(Worthington Golden),* 4 pieces 210
frozen, dinner entree *(Natural Touch),* 3-oz. patty 220
frozen, nuggets, w/rice *(Hain* Hawaiian), 10 oz. 310
frozen, roast, dinner *(Worthington),* ¾ slice 180

Vegetarian entree *(cont.)*
mix, loaf, dinner *(Loma Linda)*, ⅓ cup 90
mix, patty *(Loma Linda)*, ⅓ cup 90
Vegetarian foods, see specific listings
Venison, meat only, roasted, 4 oz. 179
Vienna sausage, canned:
original or w/barbecue sauce *(Libby's)*, 3 links 130
chicken *(Hormel)*, 2 oz. 110
chicken *(Libby's)*, 3 links 100
Vinegar, 1 tbsp.:
all varieties *(S&W)* 0
balsamic *(Pastorelli Italian Chef)* 5
red wine *(Pastorelli Italian Chef)* 2

W

FOOD AND MEASURE   **CALORIES**

Waffle, frozen, 2 pieces:
(Aunt Jemima Original) 200
(Aunt Jemima Lowfat) 160
(Downyflake Homestyle/Homestyle Low Fat) 170
apple cinnamon or blueberry *(Downyflake)* 190
blueberry *(Aunt Jemima)* 190
buttermilk *(Downyflake)* 170
cinnamon *(Aunt Jemima)* 180
oat bran *(Common Sense)* 200
oatmeal or whole grain *(Aunt Jemima)* 170
strawberry *(Eggo)* 220
Waffle mix, see "Pancake mix"
Walnut, dried, shelled:
(Diamond), ¼ cup 210
black *(Planters),* 2-oz. pkg. 340
English or Persian, 1 oz. 182
halves *(Planters),* ⅓ cup 220
halves *(Planters Gold Measure),* 2-oz. pkg. 380
pieces *(Planters),* ¼ cup 190
Walnut topping, w/syrup *(Smucker's),* 2 tbsp. 170
Water chestnuts, Chinese:
fresh *(Frieda's),* 1 tbsp., 1.1 oz. 30
canned *(La Choy/Chun King),* 2 whole or 2 tbsp. sliced . . 10
canned, sliced *(Sun Luck),* ¼ cup 15
Watercress *(Frieda's),* 1 cup, 3 oz. 10
Watermelon:
(Dole), 1/18 medium melon, 10 oz. 90
pulp *(Frieda's),* 2 cups, 10 oz. 90
Watermelon drink *(R.W. Knudsen* Cooler), 8 fl. oz. 120
Watermelon juice *(After the Fall),* 8 fl. oz. 90
Wax beans, cut:
canned *(S&W),* ½ cup 20
canned *(Stokely/Stokely* No Salt), ½ cup 20

Wax beans *(cont.)*
canned, golden *(Del Monte)*, ½ cup 20
frozen *(Seabrook)*, ⅔ cup 25
Wax gourd, boiled, drained, cubed, ½ cup 11
Welsh rarebit, frozen *(Stouffer's)*, 2.2 oz. 120
Wendy's, 1 serving:
sandwiches:
   bacon cheeseburger, Jr. 380
   Big Bacon Classic 580
   cheeseburger, Jr. or Kids' Meal 320
   cheeseburger deluxe, Jr. 360
   chicken, breaded 440
   chicken, grilled 310
   chicken, spicy 410
   chicken club 470
   hamburger, single, plain 360
   hamburger, single, w/everything 420
   hamburger, Jr. or Kids' Meal 270
sandwich components:
   American cheese 70
   American cheese, Jr. 45
   bacon, 1 slice 20
   bun, kaiser 190
   bun, sandwich 160
   burger patty, ¼ lb. 200
   burger patty, 2 oz. 100
   chicken fillet, breaded 230
   chicken fillet, grilled 110
   chicken fillet, spicy 210
   honey mustard, reduced calorie, 1 tsp. 25
   ketchup, 1 tsp. 10
   lettuce leaf, ½ tsp. mustard, or 4 pickle slices . . . 0
   mayonnaise, 1½ tsp. 30
   onion rings, 4, or 1 tomato slice 5
Fresh Stuffed Pitas, w/dressing:
   chicken, garden ranch 480
   chicken Caesar 490
   Greek, classic 440
   veggie, garden 400
chicken nuggets, 5 pieces 210

chicken nuggets, Kids', 4 pieces 170
nuggets sauces, 1 pkt:
    barbecue 45
    honey mustard 130
    spicy Buffalo wing 25
    sweet and sour 50
chili:
    small, 8 oz. 210
    large, 12 oz. 310
    cheddar cheese, shredded, 2 tbsp. 70
    saltine crackers, 2 pieces 25
baked potato:
    plain 310
    bacon and cheese 530
    broccoli and cheese 470
    cheese 570
    chili and cheese 630
    sour cream and chives 380
    sour cream or whipped margarine, 1 pkt. 60
fries:
    small, 3.2 oz. 270
    medium, 4.6 oz. 390
    Biggie, 5.6 oz. 470
salads-to-go, fresh, w/out dressing:
    deluxe garden 110
    grilled chicken 200
    grilled chicken Caesar 260
    side salad 60
    side salad, Caesar 100
    soft breadstick, 1 piece 130
    taco salad 380
    taco chips, 15 pieces 210
dressing, 2 tbsp., except as noted:
    blue cheese 180
    Caesar vinaigrette, pita, 1 tbsp. 70
    French 120
    French, fat free 35
    French, sweet red 130
    Italian, red, reduced fat/calorie 40
    Italian Caesar 150

Wendy's, dressing *(cont.)*

   ranch, *Hidden Valley* 100
   ranch, *Hidden Valley,* reduced fat/calorie 60
   ranch sauce, garden, pita, 1 tbsp. 50
   salad oil, 1 tbsp. 120
   Thousand Island 90
   wine vinegar, 1 tbsp. 0

Garden Spot salad bar:

   applesauce, 2 tbsp. 30
   bacon bits, 2 tbsp. 45
   banana & strawberry glaze, ¼ cup 30
   broccoli or cauliflower, ¼ cup 0
   cantaloupe, 1 slice 15
   carrots, ¼ cup 5
   cheese, shredded, imitation, 2 tbsp. 50
   chicken salad, 2 tbsp. 70
   cottage cheese, 2 tbsp. 30
   croutons, 2 tbsp. 25
   cucumbers or green pepper, 2 slices 0
   eggs, hard-cooked, 2 tbsp. 40
   green peas, 2 tbsp. 15
   lettuce, 1 cup 10
   mushrooms, ¼ cup 0
   orange, 2 slices 15
   Parmesan blend, grated, 2 tbsp. 70
   pasta salad, 2 tbsp. 35
   peaches, 1 slice 15
   pepperoni, 6 slices 30
   potato salad, 2 tbsp. 80
   pudding, chocolate, ¼ cup 70
   red onion, 3 rings 0
   sunflower seeds and raisins, 2 tbsp. 80
   tomato wedges, 1 piece 5
   turkey ham, diced, 2 tbsp. 50
   watermelon, 1 wedge 20

desserts:

   chocolate chip cookie, 1 piece 270
   Frosty, small 330
   Frosty, medium 440
   Frosty, large 540

hot chocolate, 6 oz. 80
Wheat, hard red, winter *(Arrowhead Mills),* ¼ cup 160
Wheat, parboiled, see "Bulgur"
Wheat, sprouted, 1 cup 214
Wheat bran (see also "Cereal"), ¼ cup:
(Arrowhead Mills) 30
(Shiloh Farms) 30
toasted *(Kretschmer)* 30
Wheat flakes *(Arrowhead Mills),* ⅓ cup 110
Wheat flour, ¼ cup:
(La Pina/All Trump) 100
all-purpose, white, bleached *(Martha White)* 110
all-purpose, white, bleached *(Pillsbury)* 110
all-purpose, white, unbleached *(Pillsbury)* 100
bread, wheat blend *(Gold Medal* Better for Bread) 110
bread, white *(Gold Medal)* 100
bread, white *(Pillsbury)* 110
cake *(Martha White)* 100
cake, white *(Betty Crocker Softasilk)* 100
gluten *(General Mills* Supreme Hygluten) 100
presifted, white *(Pillsbury* Shake & Blend) 110
white, all varieties *(Gold Medal)* 100
whole grain, stone-ground *(Arrowhead Mills)* 130
whole wheat *(Gold Medal/Robin Hood)* 90
whole wheat *(Pillsbury)* 120
Wheat germ, raw *(Arrowhead Mills),* 3 tbsp. 50
Whelk, meat only, raw, 4 oz. 156
Whipped topping, see "Cream topping"
Whiskey, see "Liquor"
Whiskey sour mixer:
bottled *(Holland House),* 4 fl. oz. 150
bottled *(Mr & Mrs T),* 4 fl. oz. 100
mix *(Bar-Tenders),* 2 pkts. 130
mix *(Bar-Tenders* Slightly Sour), 2 pkts. 120
White beans, ½ cup:
dried, boiled 125
canned *(Goya)* 80
canned, small *(S&W)* 80
canned, in tomato sauce *(Goya* Guisados) 110
White sauce mix *(Knorr),* ⅛ pkg. 25

Whitefish, meat only:
baked or broiled, 4 oz. 195
smoked, 4 oz. 122
Whiting, meat only, baked or broiled, 4 oz. 130
Wiener, see "Frankfurter"
Wild rice:
raw, cultivated *(Grey Owl)*, ¼ cup 170
cooked, 1 cup 166
Wild rice dishes, see "Rice dishes"
Wine, 1 fl. oz.:
dessert or aperitif[1] 41
dry or table[2] 25
Wine, cooking, 2 tbsp.:
all varieties, except Marsala and sherry *(Holland
    House)* 20
Marsala *(Holland House)* 35
sherry *(Holland House)* 45
Winged beans, ½ cup:
fresh, boiled, drained 12
dried, boiled 126
Wolffish, Atlantic, meat only, baked or broiled, 4 oz. . . . 139
Wonton wrapper:
(Frieda's), 4 pieces, 1 oz. 80
(Nasoya), 5 pieces 90
Worcestershire sauce, 1 tsp.:
(Lea & Perrins) 5
white wine *(Lea & Perrins)* 0
wine and pepper *(Try Me)* 0

[1] *Includes fortified wines containing more than 15% alcohol (port, sherry, vermouth, etc.).*
[2] *Includes wines containing less than 15% alcohol (burgundy, Chablis, champagne, etc.).*

FOOD AND MEASURE	CALORIES

Yam:
baked or boiled, ½ cup 79
canned or frozen, see "Sweet potato"
Yam bean tuber:
raw *(Frieda's* Jicama), ¾ cup, 3 oz. 35
boiled, drained, 4 oz. 43
Yard-long beans:
fresh *(Frieda's* Long Beans), ¾ cup, 3 oz. 40
fresh, boiled, drained, ½ cup 25
dried, boiled, ½ cup 102
Yeast, all varieties *(Fleischmann's),* ¼ tsp. 0
Yellow beans, dried, boiled, ½ cup 126
Yellow-eye beans *(Frieda's),* ½ cup 120
Yellow squash:
fresh, see "Crookneck squash"
canned *(Allens/Sunshine),* ½ cup 25
Yellowtail, meat only:
raw, 4 oz. 166
baked or broiled, 4 oz. 212
Yogurt:
plain, 8 oz., except as noted:
(*Colombo* Nonfat) 110
(*Dannon* Lowfat) 140
(*Dannon* Nonfat) 110
(*Friendship*) 150
(*Ultimate 90*) 90
(*Yoplait* Nonfat), 6 oz. 100
all flavors, 8 oz., except as noted:
(*Colombo* Light) 100
(*Dannon* Light) 100
(*Dannon* Light Duets With Fruit Topping), 6 oz. 90
(*Ultimate 90*) 90
(*Yoplait* Light), 6 oz. 90

Yogurt, all flavors *(cont.)*

(*Yoplait Trix*), 4 oz. 110
(*Yoplait Trix*), 6 oz. 160
except cherry cheesecake *(Yoplait Crunch 'n Yogurt)*, 7 oz. 140
except coconut cream pie and café au lait *(Yoplait 99% Fat Free)*, 6 oz. 180
except cookies n' cream *(Dannon Light 'n Crunchy)* . 140
all fruit flavors:
(*Dannon* Chunky Fruit), 6 oz. 110
(*Dannon* Fruit on Bottom), 8 oz. 240
(*Dannon* Fruit on Bottom Minipack), 4.4 oz. 130
(*Knudsen Cal 70)*, 6 oz. 70
(*Tropifruita)*, 6 oz. 150
(*Yoplait* 99% Fat Free), 4 oz. 120
(*Yoplait Custard Style)*, 4 oz. 120
(*Yoplait Custard Style)*, 6 oz. 190
except banana-strawberry *(Colombo Fat Free)*, 8 oz. . 200
except black cherry or lemon, creamy *(Breyers)*, 8 oz. 250
except blueberry *(Dannon Nonfat Minipack)*, 4.4 oz. . 110
banana-strawberry *(Colombo Fat Free)*, 8 oz. 220
blueberry *(Dannon Nonfat Minipack)*, 4.4 oz. 120
café au lait *(Yoplait 99% Fat Free)*, 6 oz. 170
cappuccino, all flavors *(Colombo Fat Free)*, 8 oz. 170
caramel apple cinnamon *(Dannon Double Delights)*, 6 oz. 220
caramel praline *(Dannon Double Delights)*, 6 oz. 200
cherry, black *(Breyers)*, 8 oz. 260
cherry cheesecake *(Yoplait Crunch 'n Yogurt)*, 7 oz. . . . 130
chocolate cheesecake/éclair *(Dannon Double Delights)*, 6 oz. 220
coconut cream pie *(Yoplait 99% Fat Free)*, 6 oz. 200
coffee *(Breyers)*, 8 oz. 220
coffee *(Dannon Natural Flavored)*, 8 oz. 210
cookies n' cream *(Dannon Light 'n Crunchy)*, 8 oz. 130
cranberry-raspberry *(Dannon Natural Flavored)*, 8 oz. . . 210
lemon *(Dannon Natural Flavored)*, 8 oz. 210
lemon, creamy *(Breyers)*, 8 oz. 220
lemon meringue pie *(Dannon Double Delights)*, 6 oz. . . . 180

peach *(Knudsen Free)*, 6 oz. 170
strawberry, chocolate-dip *(Dannon Double Delights)*,
  6 oz. 210
vanilla *(Breyers)*, 8 oz. 220
vanilla *(Dannon* Natural Flavored), 8 oz. 210
vanilla chocolate crunch *(Dannon Light 'n Crunchy)*,
  8 oz. 130
Yogurt, frozen, ½ cup:
all flavors:
  (Dannon Fat Free Soft) 100
  except chocolate *(Colombo* Slender Sensations) 60
  except German chocolate fudge and cookies 'n
    cream *(Colombo* Nonfat) 100
  except peanut butter *(Colombo* Lowfat) 110
  except vanilla fudge and vanilla raspberry swirl
    (Häagen-Dazs) 140
cappuccino *(Ben & Jerry's* No Fat) 140
cappuccino *(Dannon* Light Hard) 80
caramel praline crunch *(Edy's/Dreyer's* Fat Free) 100
cherry, black, vanilla swirl *(Edy's/Dreyer's* Fat Free) 80
cherry chocolate chunk *(Edy's/Dreyer's)* 110
cherry vanilla, chocolate chip *(Ben & Jerry's Cherry*
  Garcia) 170
cherry vanilla swirl *(Dannon* Light Hard) 90
chocolate *(Colombo* Slender Sensations) 70
chocolate *(Dannon* Fat Free Light) 70
chocolate *(Dannon* Light Hard) 80
chocolate *(Dannon* Lowfat Soft) 120
chocolate, German chocolate fudge *(Colombo* Nonfat) . 110
chocolate brownie chunk *(Edy's/Dreyer's)* 120
chocolate chip cookie dough *(Ben & Jerry's)* 210
chocolate fudge *(Edy's/Dreyer's* Fat Free) 100
chocolate fudge brownie *(Ben & Jerry's)* 190
chocolate silk mousse *(Edy's/Dreyer's* Fat Free) 90
coffee fudge *(Ben & Jerry's* No Fat) 140
coffee fudge sundae *(Edy's/Dreyer's* Fat Free) 100
cookie dough *(Edy's/Dreyer's)* 130
cookies and cream *(Edy's/Dreyer's)* 120
cookies 'n cream *(Colombo* Nonfat) 120
marble fudge *(Edy's/Dreyer's* Fat Free) 100

Yogurt, frozen *(cont.)*
mint chocolate fudge *(Dannon Light Hard)* 90
peach raspberry Melba *(Dannon Light Hard)* 80
peach raspberry trifle *(Ben & Jerry's)* 180
peanut butter *(Colombo Lowfat)* 120
peanut butter *(Dannon Lowfat Soft)* 120
raspberry, black, swirl *(Ben & Jerry's No Fat)* 140
raspberry sorbet 'n cream *(Edy's/Dreyer's Fat Free)* 90
strawberry cheesecake *(Dannon Light Hard)* 90
toffee crunch *(Edy's/Dreyer's Heath)* 120
toffee crunch, English *(Ben & Jerry's)* 190
vanilla *(Dannon Fat Free Light)* 70
vanilla *(Dannon Light Hard)* 80
vanilla *(Dannon Lowfat Soft)* 110
vanilla *(Edy's/Dreyer's)* 100
vanilla or vanilla chocolate swirl *(Edy's/Dreyer's Fat
   Free)* 80
vanilla fudge *(Häagen-Dazs)* 160
vanilla fudge swirl *(Ben & Jerry's No Fat)* 140
vanilla raspberry swirl *(Häagen-Dazs)* 130
vanilla raspberry truffle *(Dannon Pure Indulgence)* 150
Yogurt bar, frozen, 1 piece:
all flavors *(Starburst)* 70
cherry chocolate chip *(Ben & Jerry's Cherry Garcia)* . . . 260
chocolate almond *(Frozfruit)* 130
peach *(Frozfruit)* 100
strawberry *(Frozfruit)* 100
strawberry-banana *(Frozfruit)* 100
Yogurt cup, chocolate chip, frozen *(Breyers)*, 1 cup 230
Youngberry fruit juice *(Ceres)*, 8 fl. oz. 120
Yuca:
boiled, drained *(Frieda's)*, 4 oz. 77
frozen *(Goya)*, ½ cup 191
Ziti, see "Pasta"
Ziti entree, frozen:
(The Budget Gourmet Value Classics), 9 oz. 350
mozzarella *(Weight Watchers)*, 9 oz. 280
Zucchini, ½ cup, except as noted:
fresh, raw, baby, 1 large, 3⅛ ∞⅝ diam. 3

fresh, boiled, drained, sliced 14
canned, Italian style *(Progresso)* 50
canned, w/Italian-style tomato sauce *(Del Monte)* 30
frozen *(Seneca)*, 2/3 cup 15
frozen, sliced *(Stilwell)*, 2/3 cup 15

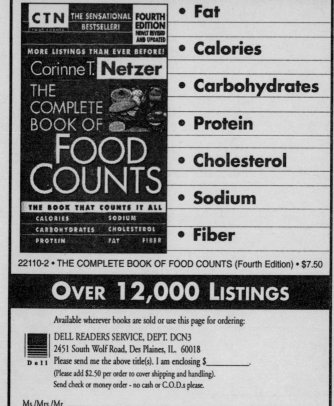

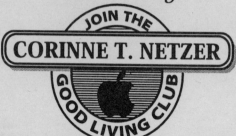